Vital Elements
24 Tissue salts and 12 trace elements

Torako Yui Homoeopathy Guide Book 5 [English version]

Vital Elements
24 Tissue salts and 12 trace elements

First Edition   25 October 2003
Author   Torako Yui
Book design   Homoeopathy Japan Co.

Published by Homoeopathic Publishing Ltd.
Homoeopathy Japan headquarters bldg.
3-49-13 Nishihara, Shibuya-ku, Tokyo, 151 0066
JAPAN <Tokyo office>
Tel. 03 5790 8707   Fax. 03 5790 8708
URL   http://www.homoeopathy-books.co.jp/
Email info@homoeopathy-books.co.jp

Printed by Panache 2000 Ltd
email: print@best-service.com

©2002/2003 Homoeopathic Publishing Ltd.

All rights reserved. No part of this publication may be reproduced, stored in a retrieval system, or transmitted in any form or by any means, electronic, mechanical, photocopying, recording or otherwise, without the prior permission of the publishers.

Contents

Introduction 6
The Next Step 8
A Case History 11
Bio elements 17
Essential trace elements 18
Vital tissue salts 21
What are vital tissue salts? 22
Directions for use 25
Examples of tissue salts use 26
Cell active tissue salts 27
Examples of cell active tissue salts use 28
Essential trace elements & environment elements remedies 29
Other trace elements remedies 30
Environment elements remedies 30
Examples of essential trace elements and environment elements remedies use 31

EXPLANATION OF MAIN ELEMENTS 32
Aluminium (Al) 33
Silver (Ag) 34
Gold (Au) 34
Boron (B) 35
Bromine (Br) 35
Calcium (Ca) 36
Chlorine (Cl) 38
Cobalt (Co) 39
Chromium (Cr) 40
Copper (Cu) 41
Fluorine (F) 42
Iron (Fe) 44
Germanium (Ge) 44
Iodine (I) 45
Potassium (K) 46
Magnesium (Mg) 47
Manganese (Mn) 49
Molybdenum (Mo) 50
Sodium (Na) 50

Nickel (Ni) 51
Osmium (Os) 51
Phosphorus (P) 52
Palladium (Pd) 52
Platina (Pt) 53
Lead (Pb) 54
Rubidium (Rb) 55
Sulphur (S) 55
Selenium (Se) 56
Silicon (Si) 57
Tin (Sn) 57
Strontium (Sr) 58
Vanadium (V) 59
Zinc (Zn) 60

MATERIA MEDICA OF 12 TISSUE SALTS 63
Calc-fluor 65
Calc-phos 67
Calc-sulph 69
Ferrum-phos 71
Kali-mur 74
Kali-phos 76
Kali-sulph 79
Mag-phos 81
Natrum-mur 83
Natrum-phos 86
Natrum-sulph 88
Silicea 90
Combination remedies of tissue salts 92

MATERIA MEDICA OF 12 CELL ACTIVE TISSUE SALTS 93
Ars-iod 94
Calc-carb 96
Cuprum-ars 98
Hepar-sulph 100
Kali-alumina-sulph 102
Kali-ars 103
Kali-brom 105

Kali-iod	108
Lithium-mur	110
Manganum-sulph	112
Natrum-bicarb	114
Zincum-mur	116

MATERIA MEDICA OF OTHER ESSENTIAL TRACE ELEMENTS 117

Borax	118
Chromium	121
Cobaltum	123
Germanium	125
Molybdenium	127
Niccolum	129
Osmium	131
Rubidium-mur	133
Selenium	135
Stannum	137
Storntium-carb	139
Vanadium	141

MATERIA MEDICA OF BIO ELEMENTS AND ENVIRONMENT ELEMENTS 143

Alumina	144
Arg-met	146
Aurum	148
Bromium	150
Chlorum-aqua	152
Cuprum	154
Flour-ac	157
Iodum	160
Manganum	163
Palladium	165
Platina	167
Plumbum	170
Zincum	172

HOMOEOPATHY INFORMATION 175

Introduction

Homoeopathy uses remedies such as vital tissue salts, cell activation salts, essential trace elements, and environment elements in order to combat the deterioration of the foods we eat in modern society (which is causing a chronic lack of minerals and leading to mineral imbalances as a result), as well as problems that stem from our intake of the wrong amounts of essential trace elements, heavy metal poisoning (which is caused by dental fillings and the environment), and problems of fluorine and chlorine.

In this book, I explain 12 vital tissue salt remedies together with 12 cell activation tissue salt remedies that support them and stimulate cell activity, as well as other remedies based on 12 trace elements, 13 bio elements, and environment elements. (Note)

Note: Institute of Homoeopathy Co. offers the groundbreaking 'Vital Elements kit', containing 12 vital tissue salts, 12 cell activation salts, and 12 trace element remedies – the first of its kind in the world.

Remedies based on vital tissue salts, cell activation salts, and trace elements heighten absorption when the body is lacking in nutrition (inorganic salts, bio trace elements), and stimulate excretion when it has too much. Homoeopathic remedies are there to give the body information and make it aware of having an imbalance. The body's natural healing ability then tries to regain the original balance. If there is a lack of something, its absorption is increased, and there is too much of something, the body stimulates its excretion. This is how the mechanism of the body works. The result is that the living body gets activated and the metabolism improves.

The first of the major factors causing an imbalance in these salts and trace elements is the existence of negative emotions, such as distress, sadness, feeling of denial, anger, jealousy, tension and anxiety. In modern-day society, we are all so busy; we never have the time to talk with each other and resolve our differences. Our relationships are becoming more complicated. If we continue in this vein, without solving the tension or anger in our relationships, we will deplete the tissue salts and essential trace elements in our bodies. The particular element, which is lacking, determines our personality. For example, when we are lacking in potassium, we become nervous and irritable, we lose our presence of mind and become stubborn. In the same way, when we became irritable, lose our presence of mind and become nervous, we use up our potassium.

Modern people are using up the energy, which they need to live at a rate five times faster than in the past. We need to train ourselves to live our lives in a more relaxed and calm manner.

A second reason for the imbalance in vital tissue salts and essential trace elements is believed to be the effect of artificial factors such as a poor environment, drugs, preservatives and hormone drugs. At the top of the list are heavy metals used in dental fillings or in antiseptics used for vaccination, which accumulate in the body and are believed to cause a variety of problems for both mind and body. There are countless people who are suffering without knowing the reason why. Environmental element remedies (note) are becoming increasingly important for people whose personalities have been changed due to the effects of heavy metals. The proper use of these remedies will enable us to live our lives with vitality as our true selves.
(Note: Environmental element remedies can be purchased from Homoeopathy Japan Co.)

1 April 2002
Torako Yui

The Next Step

The more convenient and easier life becomes, the more our health deteriorates. It seems to be difficult to develop a strong body and mind in this modern environment and with our modern-day diet.

Preservatives will remain with us as long as we regard convenience as being the most important thing. The use of agricultural chemicals will not decrease if we constantly care about the appearance of our food. As long as we dislike bacteria, chlorine will not go away. If easy mass production is what we want, there will be no decrease in the use of hormone drugs. If we don't start using public transport or going places on foot, pollution will never be curtailed. In our modern-day society, 24-hour convenience stores are taking the place of greengrocers and fishmongers and we can no longer obtain fresh and natural food. The desire to buy everything at the lowest price is causing us to lose important things. Even if something is expensive, if it is of high quality, you use it with care. Even if food is expensive, if it is fresh, locally grown produce, you eat it gratefully. I feel that such obvious, natural things have been forgotten and we have found ourselves adrift in an abnormal society obsessed with mass production and mass consumption.

Anyone preparing a family meal today is confronted by an enormous choice of food from which to select, but much of it cannot really be called food. So what is natural food? It is seasonal food grown and harvested locally. This food is the freshest and the most nutritious and is what our bodies need. In particular, we should always choose wholegrain cereal as the staple of our diet over the refined variety. This is because it is the germ that is the most important part.

White rice, white flour, white sugar, white pasta, white noodles…if these are the staple of our diet, our stomachs will pay the price. White refined foodstuff may be easy to eat and digest, but it will make our bodies lazy and our stomachs weak. As a result, we will become weak willed and lacking in fortitude.

From the outset, the very act of refining is unnatural. If we only eat refined food, from white sugar down, our digestive system will suffer. If our digestive system is not functioning properly, toxins develop in the body and our blood becomes impure. To ensure the proper functioning of our digestive system, we should eat vegetables, root crops, unpeeled fruit with the pips left in, wholegrain cereals, daikon radish and apples, etc. When I lived in the U.K. I was surprised to see my classmate eat big, sour grapes without removing the skin and pips. Since then, I have always followed her example. However, I had to stop eating watermelon seeds because I couldn't chew them properly and they gave me an ache in gallbladder.

I generally eat anything and on one occasion I ate some akebia seeds. However, I suffered from loose bowels and numbness in the mouth that lasted for three hours and was then followed by heartburn and heaviness and shrinking of the stomach. The lesson is that we should not eat things that our ancestors did not eat.

Even if we live in the centre of the city, we can still always choose natural and fresh food. The less time you spend cooking it, the more nutritious it will be. I recommend that you drink unboiled water rather than tea or hot water. Providing you can get rid of the chlorine to some extent, unboiled water makes the body stronger. Eating raw vegetables introduces a variety of bacteria into our bodies, which increases our resistance.

There are certain diets, which consist of taking only heated food and beverage. I know of one person with stomach cancer who followed such a diet. The cancer did not grow any bigger, but it penetrated much deeper and invaded his pancreas. Certain nutrients, such as neutral fats and vitamins, which are essential for the body, are destroyed by heat and it is hard work for the body to produce these nutrients itself. At the same time, I am concerned that the ability of our digestive systems to convert one substance into another and our resistance to disease is growing weaker because we are spoiling our bodies by eating only heated food. In particular, if healthy people adopt this practice in the belief that it will make them healthier, I fear that they will find it has the opposite effect. On the contrary, they may be running the danger of making themselves sick. If we pamper our bodies, they will become dependent upon such treatment. An Italian acquaintance of mine followed this method for three years. As soon as she stopped and returned to a normal diet, she developed a stomach ulcer. To do things properly requires time and perseverance. If we cook our food over a low heat, the minerals in the food will not be altered and the nutritional content will remain. However, I think it is rather difficult for people to do this nowadays.

As Hippocrates said, when we are sick we should eat raw vegetables, chewing them well. By eating fresh food, which contains the energy required for living, we purify our blood and make it much harder for sickness to occur. Fresh food retains all its original minerals and trace elements. While our meal is simmering away in the pan and we open the lid with an 'Mmmm, smells great!', the vitamins C, K, D, E and others have already gone. When we boil vegetables and drain them, we throw the minerals out with the water. Generally speaking, we should eat our food as soon as we open the lid and we should not eat food that has remained in the fridge for any more than three days. It is important to judge carefully the amount of food we are going to eat each day so as not to have leftovers. Leprosy is caused by poisoning of the intestines as a result of eating rotten food and the spreading of these toxins to the body's extremities. It is not caused by a bacterial infection. Prejudice towards people suffering from leprosy should be stamped out.

I have heard it said that, to some extent, people live longer when exposed to the severity of nature. It is important for people to get through the hot Japanese summers and cold winters without relying on air conditioning and heating if we care about our bodies. In this way we train and discipline our bodies and minds. Thus we strengthen the power of resistance of our bodies and minds. The body has been honed by conflict with the environment and its resistance is strengthened. Although we appreciate the convenience of our modern lifestyles, I believe that our vitality is constantly being dissipated. Since returning from the UK I have been living in a shabby, 40-year old house. It is extremely cold when I wake up in winter and can see my own breath, yet I am much healthier than when I lived in a house in the UK with thermostat-controlled central heating.

A Case History

Female   Age 35
Main complaints:
Infertility. She hates winter because she gets so cold. Her hands and feet are like ice, but her face is burning. She gets chilblains on her feet. She tries to take hot food and beverage and wears heavy clothing. She never eats or drinks anything cold. She urinates frequently. She suffers from poor circulation although she did not have that problem as a child. She is worn out by summer heat.

Objective view:
Her face looks a bit swollen. Her complexion is pale. Her water metabolism is poor and her body has become lazy through constant ingestion of warm food and drink. Her kidneys appear to be functioning poorly.

Yui	Do you swim in the sea in the summertime?
Patient	I never go to the sea because the summer heat wears me out. I also get a rash from the sun.
Yui	It seems like your immunity has been weakened.
Patient	Nobody likes the sun, do they? It causes skin cancer?
Yui	Who do you suppose gets skin cancer? The increase in skin cancer is due to the fact that Caucasians, who were originally from the northern hemisphere, emigrated to Australia and New Zealand in the southern hemisphere. People with yellow skin like us have lots of melanin. We won't get skin cancer from spending a little time in the sun.
Patient	I go out with sunglasses, a parasol and a long-sleeved blouse.
Yui	You have been following the wrong course. Sunlight is healing. When the sunlight is reflected from the ground into our eyes (not looking directly at the sun) it gets our body's power of resistance working and activates the body. We build a strong body and increase our resistance to colds by getting lots of sunshine and bathing in the sea. Ultraviolet rays are necessary for forming calcium.

	Although it is harmful to DNA, our self-healing powers are normally sufficient to restore any damage done. The point is that although the sun's ultraviolet rays may be harmful to the body, a very small amount of poison has a role to play in enhancing the functioning of the organism and a certain amount of sunbathing plays a role of cleansing and strengthening the organism.
Patient: Yui	But my body is so weak. I cannot start so suddenly, can I? If you do things naturally, your body will grow steadily stronger. Open the window every morning to let fresh air into the room. Eat simple, fresh food without spending lots of time and effort on it. Breathe in the air outside even if it is wet and windy. Drink unboiled water and eat fruit and vegetables in season. Cultivate a mind that doesn't fuss over small details.

Morning Night 1	Ferr-phos + Calc-phos 12X x 1 bottle (approx. 33 pillules) Ars-alb 200C x 3 days <For lack of stamina, cold body, weak kidneys, fussing over details, winter listlessness>

2wks interval

Night 2	Nat-mur 200C x 3 days <For swelling, poor water circulation, infertility, rash from the sun >

<One month later >

The patient has stopped eating extremely sweet or salty food. She feels that her body temperature has increased a little. Her appetite has increased. She has gained a little weight and her pre-menstrual irritability has decreased.

Patient	I have started to appreciate the taste of fruit in season. Previously I ate hardly any fruits because of my bad circulation. Strawberries and tangerines are really tasty, aren't they?

Yui	When you crave something sweet you should have sweet fruits. You need power to digest fructose and convert it into energy. It is not easy. But because white sugar is easily converted into energy the body leaves it there and does not bother to digest it from laziness. This also has a tendency to lead to diabetes.
Patient	Shouldn't we take sugar then?
Yui	We could not take some sugar in today's world. But we should be very careful not to take too much. We should also be wary of white, refined foods. Refined foods are no longer natural. There is nothing in nature that has been refined to become a single ingredient. Pure things are not natural for the body. On the contrary, they are toxic. Moreover, the parts that are discarded in the refinement process contain the nutrition. Brown sugar is better than white sugar. I recommend that you use naturally dried salt rather than one, which has been boiled in a cauldron.
Patient	Isn't salt also a natural substance?
Yui	Table salt is 99% sodium chloride, which is refined chemically. Magnesium is artificially added to some salts, but at the end of the day, these are artificial salts. The mineral composition of seawater is close to that of the water in our bodies. Seawater also contains other minerals. Natural salts are far more flavourful and mellow than artificial salts. In fact, when I get sick, I strip off and sunbathe for an hour and lick a lump of natural salt. I very quickly get better. If the reason for our condition lies in our surroundings, it is strange to try to get healthy only by taking remedies, isn't it? If our surroundings are at fault, then we have to change those surroundings in order to regain our health. In the Organon, the homoeopath's bible, the father of homoeopathy, Hahnemann, constantly tells us that we should breathe good quality air. He says that if we eat fresh food, avoid drugs and surgeons, and constantly correct the mind, we will not fall ill. He also said that soaking for hours in a hot spring will not cure us as it is better to take

| | a small amount of the elements contained in the spring water. However, it is not advisable to take too much of these elements. Too much is as bad as too little.
The same can be said of sunlight, alcohol, air, salt, sugar and anything. Everything should be taken in the appropriate quantity. |
|---------|---|
| Patient | To be healthy we can take vitamin A, vitamin C and other types of health food, as well as taking medicine and undergoing surgery. |
| Yui | If you want to be healthy, you should return to nature. Sadly, there are youngsters today who do not even know what is natural. In the constant quest for stimulation their tastes, their lifestyles and their sex lives are growing wilder. It is because they are getting used to stronger and more spicy junk food and cannot get satisfaction from simple food. Their tastes and their minds have grown so insensitive that they cannot appreciate the subtle tastes and delicacy of simple food. |
| Patient | That's true. There seems to be a lot more spicy food around than there used to be. |
| Yui | When I returned to Japan after living in the U.K. for 20 years, the thing that surprised me most was how hot and spicy Japanese curries are, the fact that there are so many mints and everyone drinks lots of coffee. Japan had been full of these stimulants for 20 years. I could not take any of them because they are too strong for me. I couldn't detect the subtle taste of the ingredients in food. At the same time, people spoke and behaved aggressively. There was no longer any sense of people helping each other out. People created an atmosphere of tension around them, as if to say 'it's nothing to do with me' or 'come near me and I'll kill you'. Yet when I talked to people individually, I discovered that each person had their own problems and did not know how to resolve them, so they pretended to have no feelings and feigned indifference. When I talked to them I found that they were all good people. I spend 45 minutes on consultation and I find that we are all suffering in some way. |

Patient	It would be better if we could talk frankly about our problems with our families and friends.
Yui	I think so, too. But people suppress their feelings because they think people might laugh at them or think they are strange. By suppressing our feelings we fail to understand our own lives. As a result we are unsatisfied and seek satisfaction in material stimulants.
Patient	Is it true that we tend to become irritable if we are lacking in nutrition?
Yui	That's right. For example, if we are lacking in calcium, we become fastidious and argumentative and tend towards depression. A lack of sodium causes our feelings to become suppressed and we tend to feel nothing, not knowing joy or sadness. (Refer to the following pages for details).
Patient	We have been told to take animal protein to build strong bodies. Isn't meat good for us?
Yui	Most homoeopaths tend not to eat meat. Instead we eat fish or organic chicken. If you eat plenty of beans and vegetables, including root vegetables, you don't need meat and fish. At my company we eat a cooked lunch together. Actually, 'cooked' is an exaggeration; we simply lay it out on the table. Our staples are rice mixed with 13 grains and brown rice and for the side dishes we have salad, boiled vegetables seasoned with soy sauce, pickles, small fish, fermented soybeans and cold tofu. My students and patients are surprised 'What a simple meal!', but it is enough for us. When we first moved to this building, we used to buy ready prepared meals from the shop, but we were not healthy; we suffered from heartburn and upset stomachs. Once we started to cook rice and eat mainly vegetables we became much more lively. We are no longer muddle headed or lacking in vitality. It was the oil, preservatives and spices that caused our poor condition. In a situation like that, the most important thing is to change your diet rather than taking remedies. If your environment is unnatural, it is already sick and we cannot help getting ill. The thing is that we should try not to take unnatural things

	and should exercise moderation so that we can build a healthy body which will not succumb to illness. Tissue salt remedies also have an important role to play.
Patient	I've really learnt something there. I tend to rely on external remedies without correcting my lifestyle. So what I should do when I'm feeling sluggish from a lack of nutrition is correct my diet and my mind, right?
Yui	That's right. Moreover, since tissue salt remedies and bio elements support the activity of cells in the body, such as the blood cells, bone cells and nerve cells, and combat various toxins in the body caused by poor environment, they are best used to support the nutritional balance. They are suitable for children, expectant mothers, growing youngsters, elderly people, exhausted workers and convalescents, as well as for fatigue and listlessness.

Bio elements

Bioelements, which compose human is classified roughly as it shown below;

Macroelements (Amount of the element in a body is more than 1%)
Oxygen (O)	(65%) ◎	Nitrogen (N)	(3.0%) ◎
Carbon (C)	(18%) ◎	Calcium (Ca)	(1.5%) ◎
Hydrogen (H)	(10%) ◎	Phosphorus (P)	(1.0%) ◎

Microelements (Amount of the element in a body is more than 0.01%)
Sulphur (S)	(0.25%) ◎	Chlorine (Cl)	(0.15%) ◎
Potassium/Kalium (K)	(0.20%) ◎	Magnesium (Mg)	(0.05%) ◎
Sodium/Natrium (Na)	(0.15%) ◎		

Trace elements (Amount of the element in a body is 0.0001% 0.01%)
Ferrum (Fe)	(0.0086%) ◎	Rubidium (Rb)	(0.00046%) ○
Fluorine (F)	(0.0043%) ◎	Plumbum (Pb)	(0.00017%) ○
Silicon (Si)	(0.0029%) ◎	Manganese (Mn)	(0.00014%) ◎
Zinc (Zn)	(0.0029%) ◎	Copper (Cu)	(0.00011%) ◎
Strontium (Sr)	(0.00046%)		

Ultra trace elements (Amount of the element in a body is less than 0.0001%)
Aluminium (Al)	(0.000086%) ✗	Molybdenum (Mo)	(0.000014%) ◎
Cadmium (Cd)	(0.000071%) ✗	Nickel (Ni)	(0.000014%) ◎
Tin (Sn)	(0.000029%) ○	Boron (B)	(0.000014%) ○
Barium (Ba)	(0.000024%) ✗	Chromium (Cr)	(0.0000028%) ◎
Mercury (Hg)	(0.000019%) ✗	Arsenic (As)	(0.0000028%) ○
Selenium (Se)	(0.000017%) ◎	Cobalt (Co)	(0.0000029%) ◎
Iodine (I)	(0.000016%) ◎	Vanadium (V)	(0.00000029%) ○

The rest is Bromine (Br), Germanium (Ge), Osmium (Os)

◎ Essential elements for human
○ Those elements are thought to be essential for human
✗ Those elements are thought to be mixed from surroundings into a human body and give bad effects to the body.

Essential trace elements

Hydrogen, oxygen, carbon, and nitrogen are the main constituents of protein, fat and carbohydrate and are included in the macroelements. Sodium (Na), magnesium (Mg), potassium (K), calcium (Ca), phosphorus (P), sulphur (S) and chlorine (Cl) are all included in the macroelements and microelements. These are the 11 essential elements. Sodium, magnesium, potassium, and calcium are essential metal elements and are commonly called 'minerals'.

There are more than twenty different trace elements in the human body of which twelve are recognised as essential trace elements. They are iron (Fe), fluorine (F), silicon (S), zinc (Zn), manganese (Mn), copper (Cu), selenium (Se), iodine (I), molybdenum (Mo), nickel (Ni), chromium (Cr) and cobalt (Co). In addition to these, strontium (Sr), rubidium (Rb), lead (Pb), tin (Sn), boron (B), arsenic (As), vanadium (V) and osmium (Os) are also regarded as essential trace elements. Essential trace elements are those elements that comprise less than 0.01% of our body weight and they are essential for human life even though they are present only in tiny amounts.

Trace elements are mainly constituents of enzymes. They are related to the activation of catalysts and hormones and play an important role in terms of physiological functions. As I will explain in the chapter on vital tissue salts, inorganic elements are required for organic systems to operate. Metal elements are particularly important as catalysts for chemical reactions at low energy. At the same time, trace elements serve to control the smooth functioning of our bodies. If we lack trace elements, the body functions controlled by the metal elements will not work properly.

The trace elements are so called because they control the living organism using very small traces, or amounts. Although the trace elements are good for the body, if we take them in large quantities in the form of health food or pills, as is quite common in America, it will confuse the body. So although trace elements are beneficial, taking too much is harmful. We should be especially careful with selenium, zinc and copper, as the difference between the required amount and too much is a very fine one. All the constituent elements are interconnected and if there is an imbalance in just one of the elements, all the others will be affected and the overall balance will be destroyed. Even if something is known to be beneficial to our health, taking it in excessive amounts will lead to illness.

The best way to take the trace elements is from meals. However, people's diet today is far removed from our natural diet, while our environment, too, is no longer anything like a natural environment. This has confused our bodies and they can no longer recognise what is and what is not natural. Our bodies are losing the ability to eject the unnecessary heavy metals and chemicals as well as the ability to absorb necessary minerals. In the modern world, we have countless opportunities to take in all sorts of metals through artificial nutrients or conventional medicines, as well as from our environment. We are now facing a situation in which we are not aware which elements our bodies are lacking and which elements we have in excess supply.

Half material remedies are 6X – 12X remedies which are used to obtain information rather than as supplements. Half material remedies enhance the body's ability to absorb substances it is lacking and excrete substances it has in excess. They do not harm the body and they activate the body's natural healing power. A balance of trace elements is established by the body regaining its own normal balance. The concept of supplying supplements from outside does not solve the fundamental problem. It is important that the body's self-regulating function works properly (proper self-recognition), recognising when the right amount of elements are present and enhancing absorption when the level is too low and promoting excretion when it is too high.

The appropriate amount of trace elements covers a very narrow range. Only the body knows how to control the level of elements within this range. It is the body's natural wisdom that does this. I think there are two reasons for deficiency in trace elements. One is diet. If we only eat refined products, we cannot avoid being deficient in vital minerals. This problem will be resolved only by changing our environment. The other reason is a decline in our bodies' ability to absorb the necessary substances and excrete those that are unnecessary. This problem is probably caused by the general weakness of people's digestive systems these days and by the loss of the body's natural wisdom by which it judges the correct levels of substances it requires to function properly.

The reason for the body's loss of wisdom is a blockage in the flow of the vital force.

The body's ability to absorb and excrete substances is equally balanced. When the body's power of circulation declines, its ability to absorb and excrete substances is also weakened. When a person if fixated on something or obsessed with something, the body loses its ability to excrete substances properly. When the ability to excrete properly is lost, the body's power of circulation is lost which, in turn, damages the ability to absorb substances properly. Once the flow of vital force becomes stagnated, excretion and absorption cannot proceed smoothly. The key to strengthening the body's ability to absorb and excrete is to dispel the fixation. Once you let something in, you let it go. Once you let something go, you let in other things. The important thing here is not the taking of trace element tablets, but having the right diet (having products from the sea, vegetables and grains as the main constituent and having balanced meals) and to let the body judge what is lacking and what is in surplus. Trace element remedies assist in that. The stimulation from trace element remedies is sufficient to enhance the absorption of missing elements. That also has the result of dispelling the fixation of the cells to which that element is related.

I know I am repeating myself, but it is not the material supplements that are important here. What is important is that the body is stimulated by the remedies to enable it to absorb the elements it requires and excrete the elements it does not need from the food that has been ingested. Psychologically speaking, it is releasing the fixation which is connected with that trace element.

From times past, the Japanese have eaten balanced meals, with rice as the staple accompanied by shellfish, seaweed, vegetables and beans and with soy-sauce and miso seasoning. This has become the natural meal for our bodies and I think it is important that we adhere to our ancestors' wisdom.

Vital tissue salts

1 Calc fluor (Calcium fluoride)
2 Calc phos (Calucium phosphate)
3 Calc sulph (Calcium sulphate)
4 Ferrum phos (Ferric phosphate)
5 Kali mur (Potassium chloride)
6 Kali phos (Potassium phosphate)
7 Kali sulph (Potassium sulphate)
8 Mag phos (Magnesium phosphate)
9 Nat mur (Sodium chloride)
10 Nat phos (Sodium phosphate)
11 Nat sulph (Sodium sulfate)
12 Silica (Silicon dioxide)

The followings are vital tissue salts' combination remedies.

- TS01 (Blood)
- TS02 (Hair)
- TS03 (Nail)
- TS04 (Stomach)
- TS05 (Skin)
- TS06 (Aging of skin)
- TS07 (Bedsore)
- TS08 (Migraine)
- TS09 (Sciatica)
- TS10 (Rheumatism)
- TS11 (Back pain)
- TS12 (Muscle pain)
- TS13 (Feet and leg pain)
- TS14 (Period pain)
- TS15 (Indigestion (gas))
- TS16 (Indigestion (heart burn))
- TS17 (Catarrh Sinus)
- TS18 (Hay fever)
- TS19 (Cold)
- TS20 (Irritation)
- TS21 (Bone and teeth)
- Vital salt (General)

What are vital tissue salts?

Vital tissue salts are also called simply 'tissue salts' or 'Schüßler's tissue salts' after the man who discovered them. Tissue salts were first introduced as remedies in 1875 by the German physician, Wilhelm Heinrich Schüßler (1821-1898). Schüßler believed that the body is regulated by 12 inorganic salts and that a lack in any of these salts leads to disease. Accordingly, he believed that any disease can be cured by supplementing the missing inorganic salt.

The 12 tissue salts are composed from the metal elements (Sodium(Na), Magnesium (Mg), Potassium (K), Calcium (Ca), Ferrum (Fe)) and the non-metal elements (Fluorine (F), Silicon (Si), Phosphorus (P), Sulphur (S), Chlorine (Cl)).

I regard these vital tissue salts as homoeopathic nutritious support remedies, or half material support remedies. Nutritional supplements are rarely recommended in homeopathy, but these tissue salts are the only ones recognised as providing nutritional support.

Tissue salts are normally used in potencies of 6X (10^{-6}) – 12X (10^{-12}). Judging from these dilution rates, it is obvious that they are not material supplements. The vital tissue salts are reduced to a minute level using a unique method, which draws out the latent power of the salts. After that, the latent power is released further by dilution and succussions. The amount of material is decreased in this way, but the amount of non-material information is increased. For all that, it is not like a 30C dilution in which we cannot find any of the original substances.

I use 12X (10^{-12}) potencies for vital tissue salt remedies based upon my experience. 12X could be said to be a half material potency. It is not a material potency, as when the original substance is diluted to 3X, nor is it a non-material potency as in the case of dilutions of above 12X. The material effect itself disappears at 6X and, in that sense, 12X remedies can be said to be half material remedies.

It is important to take minerals in which the body is lacking in the form of vital tissues because the 12 vital tissue salts are the natural form for the human body. Calcium supplement tablets require the body's own calcium to be digested and absorbed and there are cases where they actually invite calcium deficiency.

Vital tissue salts, which are diluted over billion-fold and succussed, retain the information of each of the tissue salts and the body absorbs the material information when the remedy is taken. The body receives the information and the stimulation and this causes the body's material recognition to begin to function properly and absorption is enhanced. The ability to absorb substances from food is also enhanced.

This is rather an extreme theory, but what we need is information not always material. The recognition of materials is performed by receptors. However, the recognition is not realised by touching each material (biologists still go under this illusion). It is recognised through the material information, which vibrates through water. Material recognition cannot take place without the water through which the vibration of the material is transferred.

The absorption of nutrients means the absorption of material information. That is the same as saying that the vital force is identical to the power to create nutrients. When the vital force flows with vigour it flows at full speed for its own purpose (its function). Under this condition, if necessary material (information) exists, that necessary material (information) will be caught (created). This is the meaning of absorption. The ability to absorb relates to the extent to which the vital force can flow without hindrance.

Taking half material and half non-material (information) vital tissue salts can enable absorption even with a weak vital force. Absorption of these vital tissue salts is related to activation of the vital force.

Even when the vital force is activated by normal remedies, if there is a lack of essential inorganic salts, the body function which is controlled by that salt will not work properly. Vital tissue salts act as lubrication for grating parts and to help the body itself function properly.

Vital tissue salts are support remedies, which promote the

smooth flowing of the vital force by supporting the basic 12 inorganic salts, which control human beings, both by means of their material information and their non-material information.

Hahnemann had already known of the importance of these inorganic salts for the human body and had researched them thoroughly before Schüßler. He remarked that the efficacy of silica, chloride, potassium chloride and calcium chloride was wonderful.

On the surface, vital tissue salts appear to be inactive sediment, yet these inorganic substances drive living organic systems. No matter how much an organic system wishes to operate, it cannot do so without inorganic salt to drive the organic system. Vital tissue salts are there to activate a static organic system by enhancing the supply and the absorption of the necessary inorganic salts.

Normally, a single remedy is prescribed for the physical and mental well-being of the patient, focusing on the patient's problem. Combined remedies are not usually prescribed. However, combinations of different vital tissue salts are known to be effective for specific problems.

If we consider remedies in potencies of 30C or higher as main remedies, those in potencies of 12X or lower can be considered support remedies. It is sometimes necessary to take support remedies over the long term.

Vital tissue salt remedies not only enhance the absorption of minerals, they also play a role in balancing the minerals in the body. If the body is lacking in vital tissue salts, the remedies encourage it to absorb them. If there is an excess of vital tissue salts, they promote excretion. The remedies are information. They enable recognition of imbalances and then the body acts to regain the original balance. If something is lacking, absorption is enhanced. If there is an excess of something, excretion is promoted. As a result, the living body is activated and the metabolism recovers.

Directions for use

When we use an ordinary remedy for a chronic condition, the vital force is shaken and tries to push out the toxicity in the body to achieve a cure (this is a favourable reaction termed 'homoeopathic aggravation'). It is because we need remedies to support this homoeopathic aggravation, and because such remedies must be safe for anyone to use, that I have introduced vital tissue salt remedies. One reason for a patient's inability to dispel his or her condition smoothly can be the patient's lack of the necessary inorganic salts. In such a case, it is important to give the patient appropriate vital tissue salt remedies.

As I mentioned earlier, there are cases in which the effect of the remedies can be enhanced by combining them as appropriate in accordance with the symptoms. However, the fundamental procedure is to take vital tissue salt remedies one at a time and wait and observe how the condition changes.

While we refer to Materia Medica for the appropriate vital tissue salt, we look for the suitable vital tissue salt based on the symptoms in the Repertory (note). If there is more than one vital tissue salt remedy listed under that symptom, you choose the one that you feel is most suitable.

If you find that a combination remedy is the most suitable for your current symptom, you can use that remedy. At the same time, if you find that one of the 12 vital tissue salt remedies seems just right for your symptom, you can use both, staggering the time of intake.

It is sometimes necessary to take support remedies over a long period of time (ordinary remedies do not need to need to be taken over a long period). Vital tissue salts are prepared in potencies of 12X and are half material remedies. However the 12X potency means a dilution of 10^{-12} (one thousand billion times). Needless to say, there is no need to worry about side effects if we take too much. These remedies can be taken by everyone, from infants up to the elderly, without worry. These vital tissue salt remedies can be used for a wide variety of cases.

Examples of tissue salts use

◇ When a remedy caused a homoeopathic aggravation (a body's reaction for getting better).

If we are suffering from chronic symptoms or are adapting unnaturally, a homoeopathic aggravation might happen. In this case, I recommend to support to push the symptom out smoothly by taking vital tissue salt remedies.

Take one conformable tissue salt remedy, and repeat depending on the degree of the symptom. Once the symptom is settled down, keep taking one or two a day for a while. If you use with 36 basic remedy kit, please take it with shifting the administration time.

◇ Acute case

Take one conformable vital tissue salt remedy (✶), then repeat according to the degree of the acuteness (every 5minutes, 20 minutes, 1hour, 2 hours….). If you take the remedy with a one from 36 basic kit, please take more than 3 – 20 minutes interval, depending on the acuteness.

✶ If the symptom does not change, please change the remedy.

◇ Chronic case

Take one conformable vital tissue salt remedy one a day for 1month to 3 months.

Example: Osteoporosis TS21 one a day x 3 months (two times a day 2 months)

If you take the remedy with another remedy, please shift the administration time.

Example: In the morning TS21 (1 bottle)

In the evening Calc-carb 30C (1 week)

◇ Constitutional problem

If you take the remedy, matching with your constitutional problems, such as bad quality of bones (TS21), bad quality of skin (TS05), bad quality of hair (TS02), bad constitutional quality (Vital salt), etc., please take it one or two a day for 1 month to 3 months.

Cell active tissue salts

Arsen Iod	Arsenic iodide	12X
Calc carb	Calcium carbonate	12X
Cuprum ars	Arsenic copper	12X
Hepar sulph	Calcium sulphide	12X
Kali alumina sulph	Potassium aluminium sulfate	12X
Kali ars	Potassium arsenate	12X
Kali brom	Potassium bromide	12X
Kali iod	Potassium iodide	12X
Lithium mur	Lithium chloride	12X
Mangan sulph	Manganise sulphate	12X
Nat bicarb	Sodium bicarbonate	12X
Zinc mur	Zinc chloride	12C

As well as Schüßler's 12 vital tissue salts, other inorganic salts known as the 12 cell activation tissue salts are also found in the body (in the tissue or blood) and they support the 12 vital tissue salts.

In homoeopathy, vital tissue salts are considered to be connected to mineral balance (a balance of sodium, potassium, magnesium and calcium) and biocontrol. Therefore, as with the vital tissue salts, an imbalance in the cell activation salts leads to illness, while blockage of the vital force leads to an imbalance in the cell activation salts.

It is important to repair the balance of cell activation salts and vital tissue salts (trace elements and mineral balance) using the 12 cell activation salt remedies and to release the blockage of vital force. Normally, cell activation salt remedies are used when vital tissue salt remedies have failed to work. Most problems are tied to an imbalance in vital tissue salts and can be treated with vital tissue salt remedies. However, when this is not the case, it will be necessary to try using cell activation salt remedies.

Examples of cell active tissue salts use

When a remedy caused a homoeopathic aggravation (a body's reaction for getting better).
If we are suffering from chronic symptoms or are adapting unnaturally, a homoeopathic aggravation might happen. In this case, I recommend to take an appropriate support remedy (vital tissue salts, cell active salts, trace elements, etc.) in order to push the symptom out smoothly.
Take one conformable tissue salt remedy, and repeat depending on the degree of the symptom. Once the symptom is settled down, keep taking one or two a day for a while. If you take another remedy as well, please take it with shifting the taking time.

- Acute case
Take one conformable remedy (✶), then repeat according to the degree of the acuteness (every 5minutes, 20 minutes, 1hour, 2 hours....). If you take the remedy with a one from 36 basic kit, please take more than 3 – 20 minutes interval, depending on the acuteness.
✶ If the symptom does not change, please change the remedy.

- Chronic case
Take one conformable remedy one a day for several weeks.
Example: Stomachache and gout
Nat-bicarb 12X x 1month (one a day)

If you take another remedy as well, please take it with shifting the administration time.
Example: In the morning Nat bicarb 12X (1 bottle)
In the evening Nat phos 30C (1 week)

Example: Suffering from full of gas with flatulent abdomen all the time
Kali-alumina-sulph 12X x 2 weeks (one a day)

Essential trace elements & environment elements remedies

Environment elements means the elements, which are feared to have mixtures from environment. They are included mixtures from dental fillings.

1. Alumina (Alminium)	Al		environment element
2. Arg met (Silver)	Ag		environment element (dental)
3. Aurum (Gold)	Au		environment element (dental)
4. Borax (Borax)	B	essential trace element	
5. Bromium (Bromine)	Br	(essential trace element)	
6. Chloraum (Chlorine)	Cl		environment element
7. Chromium (Chrome)	Cr	essential trace element	environment element
8. Cobaltum (Cobalt)	Co	essential trace element	
9. Cuprum (Copper)	Cu	essential trace element	environment element (dental)
10. Fluor (Fluorine)	F		environment element (dental)
11. Germanium (Germanium)	Ge	(essential trace element)	
12. Iodium (Iodine)	I	essential trace element	
13. Manganum (Manganise)	Mn	essential trace element	
14. Molybuden (Molybdenum)	Mo	essential trace element	
15. Niccolum (Nickel)	Ni	essential trace element	environment element (dental)
16. Osmium (Osmium)	Os	(essential trace element)	
17. Palladium (Palladium)	Pd		environment element (dental)
18. Platia (Platina)	Pt		environment element (dental)
19. Plumbum (Lead)	Pb	(essential trace element)	environment element
20. Rubidium (Rubidium)	Rb	essential trace element	
21. Selenium (Selenium)	Se	essential trace element	
22. Stannum (Stannum)	Sn	essential trace element	environment element (dental)
23. Strontium (Strontium)	St	essential trace element	
24. Vanadium (Vanadium)	V	essential trace element	
25. Zincum (Zinc)	Zn	essential trace element	

Other trace elements remedies

1. Borax (Borax)   12X
2. Cobaltum (Cobalt)   12C
3. Chromium (Chromium)   12C
4. Germanium (Germanium)   12X
5. Molybdenium (Molybdenium)   12C
6. Niccolum (Nickel)   12X
7. Osmium (Osmium)   12X
8. Rubidium-mur (Rubidium chloride)   9C
9. Selenium (Selenium)   12X
10. Stannum (Stannum)   12X
11. Strontium-carb (Strontium carbonate)   12X
12. Vanadium (Vanadium)   9C

Vital tissue salts, cell activation salts and the above 12 remedies encompass all the essential elements for a living body. Although the amounts involved are tiny, these elements are closely connected to the life systems. Naturally, we can imagine that they are closely related to our diseases.

Environment elements remedies

Alumina	(Alminium)
Arg-met	(Silver)
Aurum	(Gold)
Chlorum	(Chlorine)
Chromium	(Chrome)
Cuprum	(Copper)
Fluor acid	(Hydrofluoric acid)
Niccolum	(Nickel)
Palladium	(Palladium)
Platina	(Platina)
Plumbum	(Lead)
Stannum	(Tin)

The rest is omitted, although there are more.

Examples of essential trace elements and environment elements remedies use

- Fall of essential trace elements balance
Take a remedy for several weeks, which it seems to be lacked or surplus for self.

e.g. I feel my balance of copper is not good somehow. What can I do?
    Cuprum-ars   12X x 2 weeks (one a day)
    Cuprum   12X x 2 weeks (one a day)

- Metal element poisoning
If it is felt that a metal is accumulated in a body. Take the metal remedy for two weeks.

e.g.   Aluminium   Alumina   12X x 2 weeks (one a day)
        Lead   Plumbum   12X x 2 weeks (one a day)

Non-metal element poisoning
If it is felt that non-metal element is accumulated in a body. Take the non-metal remedies for two weeks.

e.g.   Fluorine Morning   Calc-fluor   12X x one bottle
                                                    (33 pillules) (one a day)
              Night   Fluor-acid   12X x 2 weeks (one a day)

- Dental fillings
If you have dental fillings, take the metal remedies.

e.g.   Morning   Hepar-sulph   12X x 2 weeks (one a day) for
                                                          metal in general
        Noon   Arg-met 12X x 2 weeks (one a day) for silver
        Night   Mercurius 30C x 1 week (one a day) for mercury

EXPLANATION OF MAIN ELEMENTS

Aluminium (Al)
Kali-alum-s   Alumina

Aluminium has become indispensable to our lives; it is the raw material of kitchen foil, pans and kettles, etc. Aluminium makes up 8% of the earth's crust and is contained in almost all rocks. It exists everywhere (soil, water and air) and enters the body through food, water and air. The amount present in water and air is low. Although aluminium enters the body through water or natural food, the level of intake has been growing since we started using food additives (artificial colourings, fermentation agents, preservatives, swelling agents), various medical supplies and cosmetics (toothpastes, shampoos, etc.), aluminium pans and kitchen foils. Research reveals that the average American adult takes in 3-10mg of aluminium from meals, 25-50mg from food additives, 2.5mg from aluminium cooking utensils and 1mg from tap water every day. Intake from medical supplies, cosmetics and food additives is overtaking that from aluminium cooking utensils.

The human body contains 60mg of aluminium, but the role it plays is as yet unknown. In tests on animals, aluminium deficiency has not been seen to lead to any abnormalities and is not presently considered to be an essential element for the body.

Aluminium ions have similar chemical properties to iron ions and are carried into the tissue by combining with the transferrin in blood plasma. If the body takes in too much aluminium, it will lead to weakening of the bones and atrophy and hardening of the muscles. It also accumulates in the brain and is considered to be one possible cause of Alzheimer's disease.

Homoeopathic bio element remedies work by balancing the elements (where there is a lack, they promote absorption; where there is a surplus they promote excretion). The remedies stimulate the body to begin working to regain the balance. Aluminium has become too widespread in today's world. The impression one has of the lack of lustre in the minds and bodies of people today can be regarded as a reflection of the pale, lustreless quality of aluminium. Alumina (aluminium oxide) is one of the essential remedies for people today.

Silver (Ag)
Arg-met

Silver is not an essential element and with the dental fillings and all the silver products in the world, any excess of this metal must be excreted from the body as a toxic substance.

Silver is the best conductor of heat and electricity and that is why there will always be electric currents present if silver exists with gold or other metals in the mouth. This causes migraine, mandibular ankylosis or lightning-like flashes in the head.

The effects of heavy metals (silver, mercury, copper, lead, gold, palladium, platinum, titanium, etc) on the body are serious, but the effects on the mind are far worse. We begin to lose awareness of ourselves, our character and personality changes or we may develop a split personality.

Gold (Au)
Aurum

We ingest gold from dental fillings and medicines for rheumatism or from sake (rice wine) and sweets containing gold leaf, etc. Gold dental fillings are said to be less harmful than other metal fillings and rich people have had them for centuries.

When the body contains gold, the mind and body grows hard, the sense of obligation increases or we suffer rheumatic pain which seems to pierce to the bone. It also decays the nose bone and cheek bone and encourages bone cancer.

Boron (B)
Borax

Boron is related to the metabolism of calcium, phosphorus and magnesium when there is a deficiency of vitamin B_3 and the functioning of the parathyroid hormone (related to calcium regulation). It defends against the outflow of the above-mentioned minerals from the bones and prevents osteoporosis. However, the physiological function of boron is not yet well understood.

In homoeopathy, however, the properties of the homoeopathic remedy, Borax, has been thoroughly researched by means of homoeopathic proving. In this respect, it could be said that homoeopathy is further advanced than conventional medicine.

Boron exists in the body mainly in bone, followed by the teeth, the hair, the spleen and the liver in that order. In plants, boron strengthens the cell wall and promotes cell growth.

Foods rich in boron include greenish yellow vegetables, light coloured vegetables and fruit.

Bromine (Br)
Kali-brom   Bromium

Bromine is a liquid which gives off smoke with a pungent, offensive smell. It is used for tear gas, bleach, water purification, disinfection and developing solution, etc. Bromine is used widely because of its ability to change one substance into another.

Calcium (Ca)
    Calc-fluor   Calc-phos   Calc-sulph
    Calc-carb   Hepar-sulph

It is said that the Japanese do not get enough calcium. Possible reasons for this situation could be the emission of calcium due to stress, declining intake due to deterioration in the quality of the diet, a low level of calcium in Japan's soil and water and less opportunity for exercise and exposure to sunlight.

Calcium fulfils various function in the body and calcium deficiency can lead to a wide variety of problems. When the body lacks calcium, the calcium stored in the bones starts to dissolve into the blood in order to maintain the concentration of calcium in the blood.

For growing children, the development of bone structure and teeth will be restricted, and for the elderly (particularly for women after the menopause), and sometimes even in young people, it will lead to osteoporosis.

Calcium deficiency causes back ache, stiff shoulders, osteoporosis, high blood pressure, hardening of the arteries, myocardial infarction, cerebral infarction, diabetes and gout, among other things.

Calcium also calms the central nervous system and alleviates stress. In other words, if we are lacking in calcium, we are easily affected by stress and tend to become irritable.

Milk is generally considered to be a good source of calcium. However, the rate at which calcium is absorbed is related not just to the calcium itself, but to the ratio of phosphorus and magnesium to calcium. A calcium to phosphorus ratio of 2:1 is good. In milk, the calcium to phosphorus ratio is almost equal at 10:9 and this is not considered to be a good balance.

Vitamin D is closely related to calcium absorption as a balancing factor. However, vitamin D on its own does not demonstrate this function; it becomes active vitamin D for the first time when it has undergone hydroxylation in the liver and kidneys. Vitamin D is ingested directly through food or is synthesized from provitamin D (found in abundance in shitake mushrooms) through the action of ultraviolet rays on our skin. Thus, sunshine is an equally important source of vitamin D as diet.

Calcium's rate of absorption from the intestinal tract depends upon age and other physiological factors. It is 75% in infants and 30-40% in adults. The ability to absorb calcium from the intestinal tract declines significantly in old age. (The deterioration in the calcium balance from the age of 60 is due to the decline in absorption of calcium from the intestinal tract and the increase in calcium levels in urine. The bones become desiccated and post-menopausal women are particularly prone to developing osteoporosis.)

Calcium which has not been absorbed is secreted in the stools. Calcium which has been absorbed but not used by the body is secreted in the urine or else in the stools after secretion into the intestines as bile, or is excreted in the perspiration. It is reported that exercise and stimulation of the bones is important to increase the calcium utilization rate.

If we constantly eat high-protein, low-calcium meals, there is a danger of depleting the calcium in our bodies.

We also need to be careful about our consumption of oil, sugar and phosphorus. Phosphorus is found in a variety of foods and is important for the formation of bones. However, processed food, soft drinks and instant food contain far more phosphorus than calcium and eating such foods will lead to an excessive intake of this element.

We are reported to be ingesting 5 times more oil, 10 times more sugar and 100 times more orthophosphate than 30 years ago. Excess phosphorus combines with calcium and they are discharged together, resulting in calcium deficiency. As an example, the calcium to phosphorus ratio in cola is 2:11, so we lose more calcium from the bones when we drink cola.

The balance of calcium and magnesium is also an important one. Unless we take calcium and magnesium in a 2:1 ratio, the balance of minerals is destroyed.

An adult's daily calcium requirement is said to be 600mg. Foods high in calcium include small fish, dried sardine, hijiki (edible algae) and beans.

Chlorine (Cl)
Kali-mur   **Natrum-mur**   **Lithium-mur**
Rubidium-mur   **Zincum-mur**   **Chlorum-aqua**

Chlorine is contained in gastric fluid. It activates the digestive enzyme, pepsin, and aids digestion by making the gastric fluid strongly acidic. It acts to regulate the balance of acid and alkali in the blood and to regulate the osmotic pressure of cells. It also supports liver function and is useful for removing waste from the body.

I do not think that chlorine deficiency occurs because salt (sodium chloride) is taken daily. I consider a more serious problem to be the harmful effects from drinking or exposing our skin to tap water to which chlorine is added for sterilization. In this present-day environment it is as if we are undertaking the 'proving' of chlorine.

The proving of Chlorum-aqua (a remedy made from water to which chlorine has been added) has indicated the paranoiac mentality of chlorine. Therefore, I would recommend taking Chlorum-aqua regularly to eject chlorine's toxicity.

Example: Chromium-aqua 6C   2 weeks/every 6 months

Cobalt (Co)
Cobaltum

Cobalt exists mainly in the muscles and bones, as well as in organs such as the kidneys, lungs, skin and spleen. As a constituent element of vitamin B12 and enzymes, cobalt fulfils an important organic function. Vitamin B12 is the only vitamin to contain metal. 15% of the cobalt in our bodies is contained in B12; the remainder is contained in various enzymes.

Vitamin B12 is essential for the formation of blood in the bone marrow. It is related to the formation of red blood cells and blood pigment. A cobalt deficiency can lead to malignant anaemia or a decline in muscular strength. Fatigue, lassitude, loss of appetite, dysaesthesia or neuropsychiatric symptoms can also appear.

Chromium (Cr)
Chromium

      The human body contains 2 to 10mg of chromium, but the actual content fluctuates substantially depending upon meals and environmental pollution. 60 to 70% of the chromium is combined with albumin and the remainder is combined with transferrin and carried to the organs. The highest concentration of chromium is in the lungs. This indicates that we absorb it not just through the digestive tract, but also through the respiratory tract.

      The chromium level is high in newborn babies and decreases as we grow older. This is a special characteristic of chromium as it does not happen with the other elements. (However, the amount of chromium in the lungs and fatty tissue does increase as we grow older and this is believed to be due to environmental pollution.)

      A patient whose digestive tract had been surgically removed and who was dependent upon blood transfusions developed symptoms of diabetes. When chromium was administered the patient's condition improved and it became clear that chromium is one of the essential elements for the body. It was found to be a constituent element of an enzyme connected with glycometabolism or amino acid metabolism. Diabetes, high blood pressure, hardening of the arteries and growth disorders are some of the known results of chromium deficiency. (That is not to say that chromium is effective for all diabetes.) Chromium enhances glycometabolism and enables our body to utilize energy efficiently. The result is that we gain vitality and the body's decay is prevented. It seems that elderly people tend to be lacking in chromium.

Copper (Cu)
Cuprum-ars Cuprum

After iron and zinc, copper is the third most common metal in the body. The liver, brain, heart and kidneys are known to contain a lot of copper. Copper is absorbed by the duodenum and stomach and is moved to the liver. It is contained in many enzymes and proteins and plays an important role as a catalyst in various reactions which take place in the body.

Consequently, a lack of copper can lead to anaemia, bone hypoplasia, ataxia, achromia of the hair and skin, dyskeratosis, cardiovascular problems and other conditions.

Copper enzymes are related to iron metabolism (they have the function of turning bivalent iron to trivalent iron). Copper deficiency is known to lead to anaemia which is similar to that caused by iron deficiency. Accordingly, we need to take copper as well as iron to treat anaemia.

Although copper is one of the essential elements for the body, an excess accumulation of this element can cause the development of fibrosis or cancer of the organs and is one of the causes of cirrhosis or cancer of the liver. Eliminating surplus copper is also considered to be effective in preventing cirrhosis and cancer of the liver. There is also a hypothesis that the accumulation of copper in elderly people could promote hyperoxidation of fat and lead to arteriosclerosis, arteriole fibrosis and accelerated ageing. Concerns are currently being expressed about the harmful effects of copper used in dental fillings.

It is important to get a proper balance of copper by taking Cuprum-ars or Cuprum.

Fluorine (F)
Calc-fluor   Fluor-ac

WHO (the World Health Organisation) has banned the use of fluorine (strictly speaking, sodium fluoride) on teeth as a general rule and has forbidden the use of fluorine mouthwash for children under six years of age. However, for some reason, the use of fluorine is promoted in Japan and fluorine mouthwash is endorsed for Japanese nursery school children. In Japan, fluorine is also used for expectant mothers because their lack of calcium can cause cavities, and for infants to strengthen their newly growing teeth. This policy runs counter to the world-wide current.

In the U.S.A., the incidence of cavities is said to have been reduced by the addition of fluorine to tap water. However, this has led to problems far more serious than cavities. Regarding the effect on cavities, fluorine's effect of delaying tooth eruption has been supplanted by statistical window dressing about its effect on preventing caries. There is actually some doubt as to whether fluorine really does have a direct inhibitory effect on caries.

Dental fluorosis is one harmful effect of fluorine. In this case, once a tooth has caries, fluorine makes it hard and brittle and it is common for the tooth to be extracted. Even if fluorine did prevent caries, which is considered to be its only merit, it has far more demerits.

There are far more serious problems than caries. Through the introduction of fluorine in the U.S.A. there has been a marked increase in bone cancer, osteosarcoma and the number of people with hard, brittle teeth, as well as a decline in the quality of tooth enamel. Fluorine has also been responsible for a variety of mental problems, chronic diseases, thyroid abnormalities, speckled teeth, gingivitis, kidney failure, allergies, bone deformity and under-developed teeth, among others. It has been calculated that more than 30,000 people die each year in the USA from the effects of fluorine. I, for one, would rather have caries than bone cancer.

Dean Barke, a researcher at the former US National Cancer Institute, stated that using fluorine causes cancer and that cancer leads rapidly to death. He goes on to say that this process occurs much more quickly with chlorine than with other chemicals.

Toothpastes sold at the local shop normally contain fluorine (sodium fluoride) and aluminium as an abradant. Dentists apply highly concentrated fluorine to the teeth as well as preparations composed of fluorine and silver nitrate (Arg-nit) claiming it prevents cavities. As a result, children are suffering from the effects of Arg-nit (panic syndrome) as well as becoming a Fluor-ac. type person.

I don't understand why anyone would want to use sodium fluoride, an alien substance that does not even exist in the human body and is highly toxic. In homoeopathy, to strengthen the teeth it is considered appropriate to use calcium fluoride (one of the tissue salts), a substance which exists in abundance in the body. Calc-fluor (a remedy made from calcium fluoride) is used in a bone support remedy. We are often told by patients that their teeth grew stronger after simply taking from 1 to 3 bottles of this remedy,.

As homoeopaths, we see many children with bone marrow cancer or chronic fatigue due to dissipation of energy as a result of an extreme metabolism. These children improve steadily when treated with fluorine remedies such us Fluor-acid, Calc-fluor, or Nat-fluor.

If they were not harbouring unnatural substances, they would not react to remedies with the same characteristics. It is important for parents to ascertain what is necessary for their children and what is unnecessary. The mucous membrane in the mouth easily absorbs substances directly into the bloodstream, and we should be aware that we are undermining children's health by placing alien substances into their mouths.

Iron (Fe)
Ferrum-phos

A lack of iron will lead to iron deficiency anaemia which is accompanied by palpitations, shortness of breath and loss of appetite. Since the mucous membrane loses immunity, perlèche or glossitis can occur easily. Women tend to suffer from anaemia more than men due to menstruation. If we take iron along with vitamin C or protein, it is more easily absorbed. However, taking it with phosphorus will prevent absorption.

Nori (seaweed), *hijiki* (edible algae), dried sardines and spinach all contain plenty of iron.

Germanium (Ge)
Germanium

Germanium is known to exist in the body, but its precise role has not yet been made clear. Dr. Jan Scholten, a Dutch homoeopath, is currently conducting research into this area.

Iodine (I)
Ars-iod   Kali-iod   Iodum

The body contains between 10 and 20mg of iodine, most of which is found in the thyroid gland. Iodine is a constituent of the thyroid hormone (thyroxine). Thyroxine is an extremely important hormone related to basic metabolism and growth and so iodine is indispensable for the body. Although the body only requires a small amount of iodine, only a small amount of thryoxine itself is required to control the body. Accordingly, a lack of iodine will cause major problems for the body.

Seawater contains large amounts of Iodine. In countries like Japan, where large amounts of marine products (seaweed and seafood) are eaten, lack of iodine has not generally been a problem. However, in countries where the diet is lacking in iodine, goitre is a common problem.

Although grilled sponges, containing plenty of iodine, were known to be good for goitre by 13th century alchemists, they were already in use in inland areas in ancient China. Spongia (a remedy derived from grilled sponge) is also suitable for goitre.

When iodine is in short supply, the thyroid gland grows in size in order to maintain a specific hormone level. However, if the lack of iodine continues, the gland's ability to function declines and the gland becomes greatly enlarged (goitre). Hair loss, skin disorders, physical weakness and growth disorders also occur. Pregnant woman lacking in iodine have a higher tendency towards stillbirth and miscarriage. Having too much iodine can also lead to goitre in the same way as a deficiency.

The daily requirement of Iodine is considered to be 0.1mg (100?g). It is said that the Japanese get enough iodine from their daily diet. Overseas, the daily requirement is considered to be 0.15mg (150?g) for adults. It is about the same for the European countries as well.

Iodium, Ars-iod, Kali-iod 12X work to balance the amount of iodine by heightening the absorption when it is lacking and promoting excretion when the body has too much. Of course, taking the remedy will not lead to a surplus of the element. Nutritional Iodine supplements have appeared on the market of late, but for Japanese, the danger of an excess of iodine leading to the malfunction of the thyroid gland is a greater worry. An excess of iodine is always harmful.

Seaweed such as kelp and wakame (Undaria pinnatifida) contains high levels of iodine, followed by fish and shellfish.

Potassium (K)
    Kali-mur   **Kali-phos**   **Kali-sulph**
    Kali-alum-s **Kali-ars**   **Kali-brom**
    Kali-iod

Potassium is abundant in both animal and plant life and, providing we eat a normal diet, we should not be lacking in this element. Having said that, in today's world many of us are not eating a normal diet and I believe that we are suffering from chronic potassium deficiency.

Potassium works together with sodium in neurotransmission, muscle contraction, regulation of the body's water balance (osmotic pressure), regulation of the pH level of body fluid, activation of enzymes and maintenance of heartbeat rhythm. The balance of potassium and sodium is very important and excessive salt (sodium chloride) intake will lead to an imbalance. An excess of sodium over potassium is considered to be one of the causes of high blood pressure. It also adversely affects the functioning of the nerves and muscles and causes the heart muscle to function abnormally. It also causes irregular heartbeat, heart conduction disturbance and allergies. If a person's reactions slow down and they feel powerless, it is possible that they are lacking potassium. Potassium supports the supply of oxygen to the brain and helps the mind to be clear. It also lowers blood pressure and removes internal waste from the body.

The daily requirement is 2g. Potassium is plentiful in vegetables, fruit and beans.

Magnesium (Mg)
Mag-phos

Magnesium is an essential element for us. Magnesium deficiency has been shown to increase the risk of cardiovascular disorders, particularly ischemic heart diseases (IHD) such as myocardial infarction (MI). Half of the magnesium in our body exists in the bone tissue and the remainder in the muscles and in other cells. The magnesium in the bones works with calcium and phosphorus to form the skeleton and is connected with bone growth. It also has an important role to play as a catalyst in biological reactions. Magnesium in the muscles, brain and nerves plays an important role in the transfer of stimuli between nerves and muscles, working in a cooperative or antagonistic relationship with calcium. Magnesium exists in the mitochondria in the body's cells and promotes the activity of various enzymes connected with the production of energy. It is also related to the metabolism of the nucleic acid from which DNA is formed and the formation of protein. Magnesium is an indispensable element. If there is a lack of magnesium and the level of magnesium in important organs declines, the magnesium in the bones is mobilized to maintain a constant level of the element in the fluid (the blood).

Magnesium absorbed from the intestinal tract is carried in the blood stream to tissues throughout the body. Unnecessary or surplus magnesium is discharged in the urine via the kidneys to maintain the correct level in the body.

Providing a healthy person takes normal meals, they should not have to worry about magnesium deficiency. However, a disturbance in the calcium-magnesium balance (usually due to an excess of calcium) is said to be connected to the onset or advance of ischemic heart disease (IHD) such as myocardial infarction (MI). It has actually been reported that the death rate from IHD is higher in countries where calcium intake is three to four times higher than magnesium, and lower in countries where calcium intake is less than twice that of magnesium. An imbalance of calcium and magnesium (normally too much calcium) in the blood vessel cells of arteries (cerebral arteries or coronary arteries), which send nutrition to the brain or heart, is also considered to be a possible cause of angiospasm and other conditions. It is therefore necessary to take magnesium to prevent circulatory organ disorders.

Magnesium deficiency arises not just through an imbalance between calcium and magnesium, but also through prolonged periods on a diet, which is slightly low in magnesium. Hypomagnesemia (a decline in the concentration of magnesium in serum) generally seems to be followed by some other disease. It is often seen in people with alcohol dependency or people who have taken diuretics for a long time. Whatever the case, magnesium needs to be taken with calcium in the right balance. As I have just mentioned, if we regularly take meals which give us a much lower intake of magnesium than calcium, we run a higher risk of developing diseases such as heart disease. The ideal magnesium intake is considered to be half the calcium intake. In Japan, the daily magnesium requirement for adults has been set at 300mg since 1999, which is half the daily calcium requirement of 600mg.

Foods with high magnesium content include seaweed, seeds and nuts. Dark green vegetables seem to have more magnesium than other types. There is also relatively high magnesium content in beans. There is little magnesium in animal products such as eggs or meat, so these cannot be considered as a source of the element. However, of all animal products, fish can be said to contain a relatively high amount of magnesium. Miso (fermented soybean paste) and soy sauce contain a plentiful supply of magnesium. Some magnesium is also found in drinking water.

Even when a food source contains a large amount of minerals, the more the product is processed and refined, the more minerals are lost. It is the same thing with magnesium. Refined rice contains less than half the amount of magnesium found in unpolished rice. The more refined food we eat, the less magnesium we obtain. It is known that a large amount of magnesium is lost in the cooking process (rinsing and braising). Most of the magnesium in rice is removed at the refinement stage and when washed in water, and even more is lost in the steam when it is cooked, leaving only a tiny amount remaining by the time we eat it. Although the minerals in food are not decomposed and lost through storage or heat, they are lost by washing, steaming or discarding the broth in which they have dissolved. Accordingly, we can prevent the loss of magnesium by drinking the broth.

Manganese (Mn)
Mangan-sulph   Manganum

Manganese is related to the formation of bones and cartilage and promotes bone formation. It is also closely connected with the metabolism of protein, carbohydrate and fat. Important enzymes, such as SOD (superoxide dismutase), carbonate dehydratase and hydratase, are activated by manganese.

Manganese is also closely connected with reproduction and the central nervous system. A lack of manganese can lead to a decline both in memory and in the development of the intellectual faculties. It is an essential mineral for the growth of the central nervous system (the brain and the spinal cord), reproduction and faculty development. This is why we are said to become emotionally unstable or apathetic if we are lacking in manganese.

Other symptoms of manganese deficiency which have been revealed from tests on animals are underdevelopment of the bones, the slow healing of wounds, poor synthesis of insulin or thyroid hormone, a decline in the ability to synthesize the sex hormones, malfunctioning of the sex glands, diabetes and muscular asthenia.

There is no need to worry about manganese deficiency as it is plentiful in seaweed, green and yellow vegetables, beans and eggs. However, it is advisable to note that milk prevents the absorption of this mineral.

Molybdenum (Mo)
Molybdenium

An adult's body contains about 10mg of molybdenum. It is a constituent element of enzymes involved in metabolism (of carbohydrate and fat) and the biological oxidation-reducing system (metabolism of iron). This is why it has the effect of preventing anaemia and promoting general well-being.

The liver and the adrenal glands contain a lot of molybdenum and a deficiency of this element will adversely affect the functioning of this organ and glands, which are a source of energy. That is why I call molybdenum the 'vitality element'. A lack of molybdenum can give rise to brain disorders, psychiatric disorders or abnormality in the eye's crystalline lens.

On the other hand, an excess of molybdenum promotes the excretion of copper and leads to copper deficiency disorders such as anaemia, arteriosclerosis or MI (myocardial infarction). Above all else, the correct balance is important.

Sodium (Na)
Nat-mur   **Nat-phos**   **Nat-sulph**
Nat-bicarbonicum

Sodium facilitates dissolution in the blood of calcium and other minerals and proteins and is connected with neurotransmission and muscle contraction.

Because sodium is taken as salt, we generally tend to take too much. The excessive intake of sodium is a cause of high blood pressure. If this condition worsens, we can develop cerebral apoplexy, arteriosclerosis or kidney disease. A high intake of sodium leads to a sharp decrease in potassium.

The recommended daily salt allowance for adults is less than 10g. It is a good idea to bear this in mind.

Nickel (Ni)
Nicotinum

Nickel has been used for a long time as a substrate for plating, alloys and gilding because of its silvery white sheen, the ease with which it can be processed, its resistance to rust and its low cost. However, it is easily dissolved by sweat and other substances and causes allergies.

Nickel is plentiful in bones, teeth, lungs, skin, the small intestine, the liver, the kidneys and the heart. Nickel heightens absorption of oxygen in the body and promotes the absorption of iron. It is also a constituent element of many enzymes and promotes hormonal activity and glycometabolism. Known effects of nickel deficiency are abnormal metabolism of hepatic lipids, phospholipids and glycogen, and deterioration in the reproduction mechanism. Uraemia and kidney and liver problems also result from nickel deficiency. It is possible that patients suffering from hepatocirrhosis, uraemia or kidney failure may have low levels of nickel in the blood plasma and these are potential nickel deficiency disorders.

Nickel is necessary for people who have a tendency towards metal allergies. An excess of nickel in the body is likely to be due, in most cases, to dental fillings, nickel piercings or a nickel watch strap. It is said that metal allergies, heart disease or cancer can be caused by taking too much nickel (dental fillings, in particular, cause serious problems). It is important to balance the amount of nickel in the body by heightening absorption when it is lacking and excreting the excess when a person is suffering from nickel poisoning. It should also be mentioned that, in addition to nickel, metal allergies are also easily caused by mercury, cobalt, tin and palladium. Even copper, platina, zinc and gold can cause allergies, although more rarely.

Osmium (Os)
Osmium

This is one of the heaviest of the metal elements and the hardest. Because it does not corrode, it is used for making pen nibs or watch hands. It is contained in the acervulus of the pineal gland.

Phosphorus (P)
Calc-phos   **Kali-phos**   **Mag-phos**
Nat-phos

Phosphorus is a constituent element of bones and teeth. It facilitates the metabolism of carbohydrate, stores energy and dispels tiredness by promoting the absorption of niacin.

Providing we take normal meals, we should not be lacking in phosphorus. However, if we are lacking in vitamin D, the rate of utilization of phosphorus declines. If we take in too much phosphorus, calcium stored in bones is decreased in order to maintain the balance between phosphorus and calcium, causing a calcium deficiency. It is important to have the correct balance of phosphorus and calcium.

A lack of phosphorus leads to osteomalacia, delay in calcification of the bones, underdevelopment of the bones and rickets. It is easy to take too much phosphorus from food additives or soft drinks. An excess of phosphorus can affect the functioning of the parathyroid and bone metabolism.

Palladium (Pd)
Palladium

Palladium is not an essential element for the body. It is used extensively for dental fillings and dental bridges. It is a hard metal, which does not rust and is therefore used for making electrical sockets, surgical instruments and automobile catalysts. In today's world, it is necessary to excrete these palladium poisons.

Platina (Pt)
    Platina

Platina is also not an essential element for the body. Platina is used widely for making dental fillings, artificial bones, automobile catalysts, electrical products and precision instruments. Robert Davidson, principal of the C.P.H., has said that if we were to analyse rubbish taken from outside, we would find a huge amount of fine platina particles scattered around in it. These fine platina particles in the air must surely be entering our body through our mouths and lungs. Platina is another poison, which needs to be excreted from our bodies these days.

Lead (Pb)
Plumbum

It is reported that a small amount of lead is essential for maintaining growth, as well as for reproduction and the production of blood. Lead is present in all the organs and tissues of the human body. A healthy Japanese adult contains 78 to 131 mg of lead. In a normal person, 90% of the body's lead is found in the bones. It tends to be deposited in the bones or teeth, and exists by replacing calcium in apatite (calcium phosphate).

Only about 8% of the body's lead is absorbed from food and drink. Lead absorbed by the respiratory organs enters the blood immediately, so of the 14 to 45% absorbed in this way, less than 8% is deposited in the trachea. Once lead has entered the body it combines with albumin in the blood and spreads throughout the body, finally accumulating in the bones.

Acute lead poisoning due to excessive lead intake manifests itself as colic, anaemia, nervous disorders or brain disorders. In terms of acute toxicity, lead is a comparatively weak poison and the lethal dose is 10 to 15g of soluble salt. However, lead is an accumulative poison and if it continually enters our body, even in miniscule amounts, it will lead to chronic lead poisoning. If tens of milligrammes of lead is absorbed every day, chronic symptom appear after a few weeks or months and we will experience problems with our blood, nerves or smooth muscles. As lead prevents the synthesis of haemoglobin, the haemoglobin in red blood cells decreases drastically resulting in anaemia and the patient's complexion literally takes on the colour of lead.

Leaching of lead from lead water pipes is one cause of lead poisoning, and the use of copper alloy containing lead for lead tubes and water pipes is a cause of lead pollution. The first tap water of the day contains a high concentration of lead through being in contact with it. It used to be common sense to run off the first water in the morning before using it. I wonder how many people still do that today...

Potential sources of lead poisoning include pollution from old water pipes, drain pipes, thatch materials, paint, printing presses, air pollution, lead weights discarded by fishermen, lead shotgun pellets scattered around our rivers, mountains and wetlands, and lead in fish, birds and animals that we then eat. Lead poisoning attacks the blood, causes muscle degeneration and eventually changes the personality. It suppresses the functioning of enzymes and proteins, preventing haemoglobin formation and resulting in a shortage of blood.

Rubidium (Rb)
Rubidium-mur

The adult body contains about 320mg of rubidium. As it has similar chemical properties to potassium, it tends to accumulate in the body. Tests on animals have shown rubidium to be essential for the body, but its role has not yet been made clear.

Sulphur (S)
Calc-sulph   Kali-sulph   Natrum-sulph
Hepar-sulph Kali-alum-s

Sulphur is connected with the basic metabolism of a body, working together with the vitamin B group. Most of it is present as a constituent element of proteins and amino acid. Sulphur is important for healthy hair, skin and nails. It is also important for the balance of enzymes required for brain function.

Selenium (Se)
Selenium

Selenium is known as a good mineral for cancer or as a 'rejuvenating mineral'. Tablets containing selenium are sold at drug stores as nutritional supplements.

It is certain that selenium plays an important role in the body, but it has relatively strong toxicity. The difference between the required amount of selenium and too much is very fine. Accordingly, I would not recommend taking high-concentration selenium tablets. The same is true of zinc. Taken homoeopathically, they are safe, but it is not advisable to take them as supplements. Reported effects of selenium poisoning include hair loss, nail abnormalites and nail loss, nausea, vomiting, tiredness and nervous symptoms (headache and numbness).

The soil in Finland and in the region of China running from the northeast to the southwest is very low in selenium content, and diseases relating to selenium deficiency, in particular, heart disease, are known to occur there.

Selenium plays a role in the cardiovascular system, counters low vitality and prevents high blood pressure in adults. It also acts against arteriosclerosis and thrombosis, prevents eye diseases, such as cataracts or macular degeneration, and prevents oxidation in the body.

Adult diseases, such as arteriosclerosis (heart disease caused by bad cholesterol), liver disorders, diabetes and cataracts are triggered by the large-scale generation of lipoperoxide. Selenium acts as the main constituent element of an enzyme which breaks down this lipoperoxide. It acts to reduce the lipoperoxide to prevent the above-mentioned adult diseases as well as aging and hardening of the tissues. On the other hand, it is known that vitamin E suppresses the formation of lipoperoxide and prevents its large-scale generation.

The daily selenium requirement for adults is 60?g. Foods containing selenium include shellfish, seaweed, malted rice and cereals.

Silicon (Si)
Silicea

It is known that silicon is required for the formation of calcium phosphate, which is the main constituent of bones. If silicon is lacking, there is deterioration in bone growth and skull deformity can occur. It also leads to the incomplete development of connective tissue and cartilage. A high level of silicon exists in the lungs and skin.

Tin (Sn)
Stannum

Bronze is an alloy of tin and copper and has been in use from ancient times. Tin is also used extensively in everyday objects in the form of tin plate (especially tin-plated iron) or solder (an alloy of tin and lead). It is also used for dental fillings.

Most of the tin in the body is accumulated in the bones. Tin is ingested mainly from food and water and more than 90% of it is excreted in the urine without being absorbed from the intestinal tract. Tin is considered to be one of the elements essential for mammals; tests on animals have indicated that a small amount of tin has a significant effect on growth. Of course, as is the case with other heavy metals, taking more than the required amount has been seen to result in metal poisoning. Tin poisoning disorders known to occur from normal tin compounds, not including organic tin, are acute gastroenteritis from tinned food containing high concentrations of tin and stannosis, which is a form of benign pneumonoconiosis. However, organic tin, which has been used extensively as a coating for fishing nets and ship bottoms to prevent fouling and oxidation, is deadly poisonous. In recent years it has also come to be regarded as an endocrine disruptor (environmental hormone) and the use of organic tin compounds is now strictly regulated.

Strontium (Sr)
Strontium-carb

Strontium exists mainly in the bones (the bone shaft) and, to a much lesser extent, in the soft tissues. Strontium is chemically similar in character to calcium and accumulates in the bones by replacing calcium. Accordingly, if there is an excessive amount of strontium, the amount of calcium it replaces will also be excessive. The greater the accumulation of strontium in bones, the lower the calcium content becomes, which will lead to bone degeneration.

On the other hand, too little strontium will result in bone abnormalities and increase the tendency for sprains or fractures. It will also cause deterioration in blood circulation.

Strontium with an atomic weight of 90 is a radioactive element and has become well-known following the Chernobyl nuclear power plant disaster. However, most of the strontium which occurs in nature is a safe, non-radioactive element, having an atomic weight of approx. 85. Strontium remains in the body for a long time. If radioactive strontium accumulates in the bones, it will cause bone cancer or leukaemia. That is why it is said to be one of the most dangerous of the radioactive elements.

Strontium is present in the air and is found in greater quantities in the lungs of older people than younger people. It would appear to accumulate with time. An accumulation of strontium can lead to symptoms such as rheumatism or poor blood circulation.

Vanadium (V)
Vanadium

Vanadium is a metallic element used as a pigment material for fluorescent lights and cathode-ray tubes. It is recognised and confirmed that vanadium has a beneficial effect on diabetes. Vanadium has been found to normalize blood sugar levels in patients with insulin-dependent diabetes (IDD: diabetes in which insulin is not secreted), and has attracted attention as a means of chemotherapy in place of insulin. It has also been found to normalize blood sugar levels in patients with non-insulin-dependent diabetes (NIDD: diabetes in which insulin is secreted, but insulin sensitivity is reduced due to stress or obesity). However, the mechanism involved has not yet been made clear.

Vanadium is involved in fat metabolism and acts to maintain the neutral fats. It is related to fatty liver and fatty heart. It also increases glycogen storage in the liver and promotes glucose utilization in the muscles. It is also known to support the growth of bones and teeth. It also aids cell regeneration together with zinc and supports iron metabolism and blood formation.

Sea squirts are rich in vanadium, although, for me, they are creepy looking things. Other foods high in vanadium are edible algae, seaweed and shellfish. Spriing water from Mt. Fuji has a high concentration of vanadium and is known as being good for diabetes.

Zinc (Zn)
Zincum-mur   Zincum

Zinc is the second most common metallic element found in the body after iron. Most of it exists in tissue cells combined with protein, and predominantly in large tissue cells such as the muscles, bones and skin. Although it exists in considerably high concentration in the liver, pancreas, kidneys and brain, its concentration in the prostate and bones is particularly high. In fact, zinc is closely connected with reproduction and bone formation. Skin disorders are the main signs to appear when the body is lacking in zinc.

Chemical reactions in a living body are realized by enzymes. Certain enzymes require metallic elements, and zinc is one such element, which works to activate enzymes. Magnesium, iron and copper are the main metallic elements, which activate enzymes. There are many enzymes, which need zinc. If zinc is lacking, it affects metabolism and give rise to a variety of problems for the body. It is also a constituent element of various hormones such as insulin and is connected with the action of hormones and the adjustment of hormonal secretion.

      Zinc deficiency is known to cause the following conditions.

(1)   Growth inhibition and dysgeusia (taste blindness, becoming insensitive to subtle salt tastes).

It is known that growth is inhibited if zinc is lacking. One of the reasons for this is that dysgeusia occurs, which suppresses the appetite and leads to lower food intake. As a result of the dysgeusia, the absorption rate declines. This is true of anything; if we do not eat food with great relish, we will not gain nutrition from it. In this way, zinc deficiency sometimes arises in people who are insensitive to taste and in children whose appetite is low or whose growth is poor. There is also a possibility of zinc deficiency arising in adults who have become insensitive to taste. Another major reason for growth inhibition and dysgeusia is the fact that zinc is needed for the formation of nucleic acid. As nucleic acid is a constituent element of genes, it is an essential element for an organism which undergoes metabolism and particularly so during the period of growth.

Although it is not known why dysgeusia and loss of appetite should occur, we can assume that zinc is closely connected with the transmission of the information pertaining to the sense of taste, since it is found in the taste buds and in saliva.

(2) Deterioration in metabolism of skin and bones
Hyperkeratosis and slow healing of wounds on the skin are known to occur when zinc is lacking. The connective tissue in skin and bones contains a large number of fibrous proteins called 'collagen'. Zinc is considered to be connected with the synthesis of collagen. It is also known that zinc acts to promote bone formation.

(3) Delay in sexual maturity in both sexes. Decline of the generative function in both sexes.
Zinc deficiency inhibits the formation of spermatozoons and ova, and sexual dysfunction occurs. Zinc is considered to be connected with reproduction.

(4) Prostate disorder (dysuria, feeling of residual urine, incontinence, etc.)

(5) Diabetes (zinc is also connected with insulin production in the pancreas.)

(6) High blood pressure, arteriosclerosis, dementia and cancer

(7) Sense of smell disorders

(8) Underdevelopment in the fetus (in particular, brain underdevelopment and reduced immunity.)

(9) Underdevelopment in infants (in particular, genitalia underdevelopment, immunity deficiency, and brain underdevelopment.)

(10) Skin disorders (zinc is also connected with the formation of collagen.)

(11) Immunity disorders (zinc is also connected with lymphocytes, which control immunity, and enhancement of the T-cells' function. Infections occur easily when zinc is lacking.)

(12) Decline in ability of wounds to heal.

(13) Hair loss and wide adverse effect on mental activity
Taste disorders and loss of appetite are early symptoms of zinc deficiency. Other symptoms to appear are underdevelopment and diarrhoea along with specific skin symptoms (inflammation). Zinc deficiency can arise when our diet is extremely low in zinc or we take a large amount of a substance, which prevents its absorption (some

medicines are known to react chemically with zinc and prevent its absorption). Zinc taken from food is absorbed through the intestinal wall. The absorbed zinc enters the blood stream and combines with the proteins called albumin and globulin, and is carried to the tissues. Zinc which has been used and is no longer required is for the most part excreted in the stools and to a lesser extent in the sweat and urine. When the body lacks zinc, its absorption from the intestinal tract is enhanced. The average absorption rate of zinc contained in food is about 60%. This figure will be markedly different for a healthy person and someone with an intestinal disorder.

Dietary fibres, calcium and metals such as copper or cadmium are said to prevent the absorption of zinc. Foods containing zinc include oysters and other seafood, sesame seeds, beans, meat, clams, soybeans and unpolished rice.

MATERIA MEDICA OF 12 TISSUE SALTS

I would like to introduce materia medica of 12 vital tissue salt.

NOTE
<Mind> is mental pictures of the remedy.
<Special Characteristics> is peculiar characters of the remedy.
<Region> is related organs or parts with the remedy
<Modality> 'Worse' indicates when the person gets worse.
For example, Calc-fluor is the remedy for a person, who gets an illness by a first move or chillness.
On the contrary, 'Better' indicates when the person gets better.
For example, Calc-fluor is the remedy for a person, who gets better by continuous move or warmth.

By using above information, we choose a remedy, which seems the most suitable for a problem.

Calc-fluor
Calc-f.

<Mind>	Deep depression
		Fear of losing money
		Stinginess
		Not realistic/not practical
		Indecisive. Difficult to judge.
		Value on money rather than on a human being

<Special Characteristics>
		Restless
		Body is cold
		Lack in elasticity of tissue and vessels
		Lost of elasticity of skin (easy to have wrinkles)
		Haemorrhage in uterus
		Brittle bones and teeth, caries
		Problems of bones and teeth (lack of enamel in teeth, easy to have a decayed tooth)
		<u>Diseases due to tense and stretch too much in ligaments, muscles, joints</u>
		ganglion
		Swell in lymphatic glands
		Droop in bladder or abdomen

<Pregnancy>	This remedy makes a delivery to go well during labour
		Problems in a fetus' bones
		Weak labour pain
		Induration of glands (the tonsils, the mammary gland, hemorrhoid, tumour)
		Constipation (due to relaxation of rectum's muscles)
<Region>	Periost, Vein, Artery, Glands, Muscle, Skin, Left side
<Modalities>
Worse		First movement, Chill, Dampness, Draft,
		Change of weather, Sprain
Better		Continuous movement, Warmth, Rub, Cold compress

Calc-fluor: Case

11 years old   Boy
Main complaints: Hard ganglion in his wrist

It was much watery one year ago, and was taken out by an injection. However, it has been swollen again, and it seems that the bone is hard and deformed.

Yui   'How are his teeth?'
Mother 'They are relatively strong, but he tells me that they ache if he eats sweets and cold things.'
Yui   'How about your own teeth?'
Mother 'They are weak. Before I got pregnant, I was advised to apply fluorine to make them to be strong, and I did so. I don't tend to have decayed teeth so much since then.'
Yui   'When he was born, did anything wrong thing happen?'
Mother 'In fact, he had a harelip slightly. He had operation immediately, so he escaped with having a small scare only.'
        *Calc-fluor is a remedy for a harelip and ganglion.
Yui   'What would you like to be in future?'
Boy   'As I am good at mathematics, I would like to use this talent.'
Mother 'He is a capable person, and saves a New Year's gift (money) and his pocket money a lot. I was also a tightfisted person comparatively. '

Calc-fluor 12X 1 bottle (approx. 33 pillules) x Morning and Night

After one month, the ganglion had been getting smaller.

Night 1   Calc-fluor 1M x 2 days

Two weeks interval
Night 2   Ruta 10M x 2 days

After three months, ganglion had disappeared, and discharges from his ears had been dried. Surprisingly, his deep attachment to money has been also decreased, and he bought a stuffed toy as a present to his sister.

Calc-phos
Calc-p.

<Mind>　　　　Being forgetful badly
　　　　　　　Cannot think (due to tiredness) Children, whose thinking power is low
　　　　　　　Anxiety
　　　　　　　Cries easily, difficult, and vacant child
　　　　　　　Too much use of brain, disappointment, sadness makes everything worse

<Special Characteristics>
　　　　　　　Dissatisfaction (desire for change and travel)
　　　　　　　Sigh
　　　　　　　Lack of enthusiasm, dull mind
　　　　　　　<u>The most suitable to problems of a growth phase (grow too rapidly or being small extraordinary)</u>
　　　　　　　Growth pain
　　　　　　　Problems in bones and teeth (weak teeth, osteoporosis)
　　　　　　　Indigestion (potassium metabolism is weak and often have indigestion)
　　　　　　　Albuminuria
　　　　　　　Anaemia children, anaemia in youth (esp. in a growth phase)
　　　　　　　Too thin
　　　　　　　Frostbite
　　　　　　　Problems in lymphatic glands
　　　　　　　Difficulties in healing symptoms
　　　　　　　Easy to be tired
　　　　　　　Too much leucorrhoea and heavy flow in period
　　　　　　　Chronic pneumonia
　　　　　　　Tuberculosis of intestines diarrhea
　　　　　　　Tuberculosis of lungs and profuse sweat at night
　　　　　　　Easily to have polyps

<Pregnancy> Mastitis
A baby does not drink mother's milk, as it is salty
Bad quality of mother's milk
Pain in bones of limbs during pregnancy
Tiredness after labour

<Region> Bone, Sutures, Periosteum, Cartilage, Glands, Nerves, Abdomen, Chest

<Modalities>
Worse   Change of weather, Draft, Cold air, Dampness, Thawing, East wind, Teething
Better Summer, Warm dry air, Lie down

Calc-phos: Case

12 years old   Boy
Main complaints: Pain in growth

- Pain in joints of elbows and knees. They sometimes cramp.
- Not so much appetite, considering how fast his height grew. Always eats junk food
- Cannot get up in the morning. Vacant.
- Sleepy during classes. Teachers warned him, but he cannot concentrate on and feel dull all over his body.
- Easily takes cold
- Easily gets an injury. He broke a bone just because he fell over.

Calc-phos 12X 1bottle (approx. 33 pillules) x Morning and Night

Calc-phos suits to quality of bones, bone growth, and problems of lymphatic glands.
It also suits to anaemia, and becomes nutrition for bone and blood by using together with Ferrum-phos. It is important to use for a growth phase, osteoprosis, anaemia, and pregnancy's problems.

Calc-sulph
Calc-s.

<Mind> Unsettled emotion
Changeable mind
Suddenly forget things, although he/she has conscious
His/her mind is not at present due to anxiety and irritation
Many grumbles and dissatisfactions
Lots of fears

<Special Characteristics>
The third stage of inflammation (suppurative discharges)
Body is warm (influenced by both of hot and cold temperature)
A composition substance of blood
Lack of blood coagulation
Acne in youth
Toxins in a body
Dermatitis, which is difficult to heal
Dried lips
Abscesses and boils. They are easily suppurated
Ulcer
Problems in liver
Chronic rheumatism, which is better for cold
Suppurative discharges
<u>Constant yellow pus discharges</u>
Suppurative discharges due to ulcers or tumours in intestines
Inflammation in connective tissue
Ulcers in eyes
Mastitis (Pus)

<Face> Gerontal macula (aging mark), which looks dirty,
Liver spot, Yellowish

<Region>　　　Connective tissues, Glands, Mucus Membrane, Bones, Skin

<Modalities>
Worse　　　Draft, Warmth, Cold, Wet
Better　　　Fresh air, Open air, Bath
Calc-sulph: Case

8 years old Boy
Main complaints: Abscess

- Easily gets abscess, which tends to be festered
- Easily gets frostbites, from where starts to have ulcers and bleed and have pus
- Easily gets conjunctivitis, which tend to have pus

Morning	Calc-sulph 12X	x 1bottle (approx. 33 pillules)
Night 1	Hepar-sulph 12X	x 2 weeks
Night 2	Hepar-sulph 200C	x 2 days

Calc-sulph has a character, which forms pus, and it is similar to Silica and Kali-sulph.
It suits to connective tissues and is used for children, whose arms tend to dislocate.

Ferrum-phos
Ferr-p.

<Mind> Feels normal things as abnormal things
Looses bravery and hope (Slightly better after sleep)
Takes as a big thing, although it is a trivial thing
Delusion due to congestion in brain
Paranoiac feelings
Extremely talkative
Irritable
Dizziness from anger or congestion in head

<Special Characteristics>
All of the early stage of inflammation (=Aconite)
The first stage of inflammation
Complaints after surgery
Hearing problems due to taking cold
Lost in muscle tension
Lost in muscle firmness (due to widen vessels and skin gets itchy)
Itchiness in skin
Oxidation of blood
Respiratory organs disorders
Imbalance of iron in a body
Tends to have a ruddy face
Anaemia
Frostbites
Fresh wounds due to accident or injury
Hemorrhage from hemorrhoid

<Pregnancy> Anaemia in pregnancy
Morning sickness. She vomits everything she ate
Fever during pregnancy
Childbed fever after labour

<Face> Red cheek and forehead. Especially, when he/she has inflammation orafter a little exercise. Black rings

<Region>	around eyes Circulations (lungs, ears, nose), Vessels, Blood, Heart, Brain, Mucus membrane, Bones
<Modalities>	
Worse	Night, Noise, Creaked sound, Suppression of perspiration, Physical exhaustion
Better	Cold, Hemorrhage

Ferrum-phos: Case

1. 8 years old   Girl
Main complaints: High fever due to taking cold

- She looked fine, as her face was red, flush and shiny.
- Took Belladonna, but no change
- Started to cough with having ear ache
- She tends to have nosebleed. When she has fever, the nosebleed does not stop.

Ferrum-phos 12X   Repeat every one hour

Ferrum-phos suits all of the early stage of inflammation
It also suits tympanitis, so it works better for otitis by using it with Kali-mur.

2. 28 years old   Female
Main complaints: Anaemia

- Has dizziness and nausea when her period starts
- Easily get flush. When she becomes nervous, even it is the slightest degree, she becomes red.
- Having inflammation in her throat, tends to cough
- Easily gets tired
- Hates eggs

Morning	Ferrum-phos 12X	x 2 bottles (aprox. 66 pillules)
Night 1	China 6C	x 10 days
Night 2	China 200C	x 2 days

Ferrum-phos suits haemoglobin insufficiency and oxygen insufficiency. It plays a role of purifying blood by being used for inflammatory problems.
China works for problems in liver and spleen. They regain their original function and purify blood by given it. Those two remedies suit anaemia. Try Ferrum-phos for anaemia during pregnancy.

Kali-mur
Kali-m.

<Mind>	Dissatisfaction and discouragement
	Fear of evil
	Being quiet and still
	Wonders if he/she dies from hunger
	Irritation and anger for trivial things

<Special Characteristics>
	Whitish, adhesive and thick discharges
	Phlegmatic ears, Hearing problems due to otosalpinx catarrh
	Tonsillitis 'White membranes in tonsils'
	The second stage of inflammation (Anti-inflammation for the middle)
	For harmful effect of vaccination
	Milky moss on tongue
	Milky colour discharges
	Swelling in glands (tonsil, parotid gland)
	<u>No. 1 remedy for swellings in lymphatic gland</u>
	Inflammation in connective tissue and swell
	Whitish stool after diarrhea (also whitish urine)
	Slight problem in respiratory organs
	Cough
	Symptoms of cold
	Ear diseases, full of discharges, starts not to be able to hear
	Children's cold with fever

<Pregnancy>	Morning sickness with vomiting white gastric fluid
	No.1 remedy of childbed fever
	Swellings in breasts

<Region>	Epitheliums (throat, otosalpinx), Mucous glands, Occiput, Muscles, Left side
<Modality>
Worse	Fresh air, Cold drink, Fat, Rich food

Kali-mur: Case

9 years old Girl
Main complaints: Blockage in otosalpinx

- Whitish ear wax has been accumulated in her ears. Tends to have difficulty in hearing.
- When it is dried, it sounds like leaves' rubbing sound. It annoys her.
- She does an earpic (cleaning her ears) every day
- She has been having nasal congestion for a long time. She takes a medicine for changing her constitution, which decreases her mucous.
- She took all kind of vaccination
- She tends to take cold
- She is small

Morning	Kali-mur 12X x	1 bottle (aprox. 33 pillules)
Night 1	Vaccininum 200C x	2 days One week interval
Night 2	Pulsatilla 200C x	2 days

This case covers every symptoms of Kali-mur, however there are harmful effects of vaccination and a medicine, which she has taken. As they have put a lid of her symptoms, I prescribed remedies for these problems (Night 1 and 2). Those remedies would help to push her symptoms smoothly. (*I was reported that she has started not to take the medicine so much.)

After one month, she took cold, having greenish nose discharge and much more discharges from her ears, but all was completely cured. As other changes, she has started to have stamina and become active, although she did not have physical strength and was weak. The amount of her ear wax has been decreased, and she does an earpic (cleaning her ears) once a week now.

Kali-mur 12X x 1 bottle (approx. 33 pillules)
She is now growing a lot without taking cold.

Kali-phos
Kali-p.

<Mind>   Very nervous and anxiety
Irritable
Gloomy feeling, negative thinking
Does not like works or rules
Does not associate with people
Force of going the opposite direction
Vacant due to too much mental exertion
No patience
Extremely forgetful (curtails words in a sentence)
Sensitive to sounds, and does not like music
Does not have energy, and easily gets tired
Indecisive and changeable
Cannot get out from fears and agonies
Hallucinations
Going mad
Homesick
Melancholy
Hysteric, and laughs with crying
Cannot suppress feelings
Depression and sigh
Worries about own diseases
Shy and tends to become red
Insomnia
Suspicious

<Special Characteristics>
<u>Mental exhaustion, Nervous breakdown</u>
Asthenia and weakness
Extremely exhausted both in mental and physical
Indigestion from neurosis
Headaches due to mental disorder
Easily gets excited
Marked characteristic of changing a constitution to alkaline

Bright yellow or orange yellow discharges
Offensive discharges (rotten onion)
Sensitive to sound and headache in occiput
Suspicious and tends to be homesick
Weak in motor nerves, tends to have convulsions
Convulsions in whole body
Anaemia
Bald
Ganglion

<Pregnancy>	Tendency of miscarriage due to being neurotic
	Tiredness and fatigue after labour
<Face>	Grey or pale, dirty look as he/she did not wash the face
<Region>	Nerves (brain; spinal cord), Excretion, Mucus membrane, Skin, One side
<Modality>	
Worse	Worry, Exhaustion, Pain, Cold and dry air, Adolescence
Better	Eating, Light movement

Kali-phos: Case

18 years old   Male
Main complaints: Problems before entry examination of university

- Mental fatigue
- Too much mental exertion
- Lack of sleep
- There are so many things to remember, but the more he is hasty, the less he memorises.
- He has started to get cold sweat, cannot relax.
- 'I cannot pass, if I am like this!' depressed and closed
- Feels paralysed in muscle, heavy and dull
- Cannot sleep

Morning	Kali-phos 12X	x	one bottle (33 pillules)
Night 1	Gelsemium 6C	x	10 days
Night 2	Gelsemium 200C	x	2 days

Kali-phos suits nerves, especially the central nerves and the autonomous nerves. If Kali-phos is lacked, intellectual and mental abilities are fallen, and the person gets depression.

It also suits brain's fatigue. In this case, this person gets autonomic imbalance (vegetative dystonia) by overtaxing his/her brains repeatedly or repeated anxieties. If this condition continues, the quality of blood gets worse and sometimes gets leukaemia. Kali-phos also suits leukaemia. It is needed to people, who undergo dialysis, as well.

Kali-sulph
Kali-s.

<Mind>
Fear of falling from top
Very irritable
Anxiety in the evening
Worse from using mind
Always in hurry
Shy
Obstinate and selfish
Indolent and lazy

<Special Characteristics>
The third stage of inflammation (Festered eruption, acne, yellow or green
mucus, Nasosinusitis, discharges from ear, catarrh, hepatitis, nephritis, etc)
Body is warm (cold limbs)
(Sticky) <u>Profuse yellowish discharges</u>
Plays a role of carrying oxygen as well as iron
Adjusting skin
Inflammation of skin
Develops dandruff easily, and inflammation of scalp
Red, sore, and itchy skin with yellow discharges (atopic eczema)
Fragile nails
Melanoma
Chronic rheumatism
The late stage of inflammation
Does not like warm room
Likes cold of fresh air

<Face> Yellow to brownish complexion, Freckles, Pigment composure, Discolorationed skin
<Region> Epithelium (Respiratory organs, skins), Glands

<Modality>
Worse   Warmth, Eggs
Better   Cool

Kali-sulph: Case

8 years old   Girl
Main complaints: Atopic eczema

- Yellow discharges
- Tears, when it gets warm and the condition gets worse
- Applied cortisone cream, when she had bad lacquer poisoning before she had atopic eczema
- Shy and does not like people
- Always irritable
- Discharges from ears, or eye mucus, everything is yellowish and is purulent
- Also has bronchitis, phlegm is also yellow

Morning	Kali-sulph 12X	x	one bottle (33 pillules)
Night	Petroleum 6C	x	two weeks

Kali-sulph suits problems in epithelium. It is also used for the case, which the symptom does not progress and cannot be pushed out.

Mag-phos
Mag-p.

<Mind> Dislike to think accurately, forgetful
Sulky and feels sad
Grief for pain with having hiccups
Always talking to himself/herself or sitting sullen without saying anything
Keeps changing objects' place from here to there
Feels fatigue much mentally and physically

<Special Characteristics>
Sensitive and nervous
Impulsive and extreme
Symptoms in right side (head, ear, face, chest, ovaries, and sciatica)
Worse from chill
Better from warmth
Convulsion or cramp in muscles
Colic (Better from pressure)
Gas in abdomen, inflated abdomen
Cramp in legs
<u>General pains and period pain</u>
Thin and slim person, who has nervous temperament
(Kali-phos is for mental or nervous fatigue, Mag-phos has nervous
temperament with physical symptoms)

<Pregnancy> Pain as cramp during labour
Cramp in legs, followed by convulsive pain
Separation of the placenta

<Region> Nerves, Muscles, Right side

<Modality>
Worse Chill, Draft, Cold water, Touch, Periodical, Night, Extreme exhaustion
Better Warmth, Hot bath, Pressure

Mag-phos: Case

45 years old Male
Main complaints: Cramps and pains in leg muscles

- Swelling feeling in abdomen and colic after meals
- Pains everywhere in his body, always complaining
- Tendons in fingers cramp when he writes
- Utterly exhausted mentally and physically due to pains
- He wonders if he is sensitive as the pains are so extreme
- Only when he takes bath and gets warm, the pains are relieved

Mag-phos 12X x one bottle (approx. 33 pillules) Morning and Night

Magnesium suits problems in muscles. Phosphorus suits problems in nerves. Consequently, Mag-phos suits convulsion symptoms. It is the most suitable to pains.

Natrum-mur
Nat-m.

<Mind> Despair (especially about future)
Does not like sympathy
Discouraged soul
Feelings come to heart
Strong sense of responsibility
Always remembers unpleasant things in the past
Tears nearly burst, but does not cry
Difficult to be pleased
Constipation
Wants to sing and dance
Fearful
Adolescent depression
Vacant mind
Easily gets hurt
Fear of being rejected

<Special Characteristics>
Craves for salts
Distribution and circulation of water in a body
Swellings in a body
Takes cold with tears and nasal mucus (watery)
Watery and whitish discharges
Cannot taste and smell due to hay fever
Malnutrition
Thin even he/she eats a lot
Anaemia
Deterioration of heart function and thyroid glands function
Chronic pain in throat
Headache in frontal lobe (Worse in morning)
No hope and despair
Depression
Bald
Develops dandruff easily

<Pregnancy>	Skin symptom with blisters Herpes Zoster
<Pregnancy>	Morning sickness Swellings Vomit whitish mucus Falls hair during labour or breast feeding
<Region>	Mind, Heart, Mucus glands, Spleen, Liver, Intestines, Skin

<Modality>
Worse   Periodically, Heat (Sun, Summer), Sympathy, Adolescence, Seaside
Better   Fresh air, Perspiration, Seaside

Natrum-mur: Case

33 years old Femal
Main complaints: Problems in feelings during pregnancy

- The 6th month of being pregnant (she was blessed a baby at last)
- Swellings (Especially bottom parts)
- Tends to have vesicles in hands and around mouth
- Maudlin
- Easily gets angry
- Very moody, feels her husband finds her unmanageable
- Headache in frontal lobe in the morning
- Hates eating
- Cannot smell
- Her pubic hair fell, and her hair has also become to fall easily
- Worries if she can bring a baby up after the birth

Morning   Nat-mur 12X x   one bottle (approx. 33 pillules)
Night   Nat-mur 30C x   one week
Nat-mur suits problems in fluid balance in a point of tissue salts. She

has swellings and seems to have herpes.
She has also become moody due to the heighten function of thyroid. Nat-mur suits such problems, as well. I prescribed her Nat-mur 30C at night as an intension of curing her mental problem (inner child), which has not been sorted out yet. I could have prescribed 200C, but chose 30C to move her vital force gently, as she is at her pregnancy.

Natrum-phos
Nat-p.

<Mind> Fear with imagining something bad happens
Anxiety
No purpose
Forgetful
Lack of thinking power
Sees furniture as a human (still half-sleep), and can hear human's voices
Nervous temperament
Cares about trivial things

<Special Characteristics>
Craves for deep fried food and rich taste
Sour smell, sour taste, hyperchlorhydria, belch
Heartburn
Indigestion in stomach
<u>Secretion of gastric fluid</u>
Yellow discharges
Stiffness after moderate activity
Ejaculation every night
Green stool, when he/she has diarrhea
Rheumatism
Abnormal lactic acid in babies (It is normally due to too much breast feedings)
Pale yellow moulded like in tongue
Pain worse from thunder
Jaundice
Itchy all over body
Abnormality in thyroid glands

<Pregnancy> Morning sickness. She vomits gastric fluid

<Region> Occiput, Mucus membrane, Duodenum, Gallbladder, Genitals, Nerves, Stomach, Intestines

<Modality>
Worse   Sugar, Infant, Ejaculation, Period, Sour food
Better   Chill, Fresh air

Narum-phos: Case

35 years old Femal
Main complaints: Cholecystitis and gallstone

- Cannot eat boiled eggs
- Too much gastric fluid
- When she eats fatty food, she has indigestion
- Yellow moss on her tongue
- Food and water remains in her abdomen, being able to hear the water move from there
- Constipation alternates with diarrhea
- Her stool smells sour, when she is diarrhea
- Arthritis in toes, which is painful
- She imagines a lot, when she goes to bed. 'Is somebody next to me?' ' Will I have a burglar?', etc. and cannot sleep.

Nat-phos 12X x   two bottles (66 pillules) Morning and Night

Nat-phos is good for the case, which a body cannot excrete fat, and forms soft fat at side, chests, and groins (tubercle formation). As a result, it occurs chronic rheumatism, and the pain gets violent due to the acid constitution.

Natrum-sulph
Nat-s.

<Mind> Suicidal thinking
Needs a rest, but cannot sleep at night due to being irritable
Depression from listening to music
Depression or suicidal desire since he/she hit a head
Tends to hit head
Packs other's agony and own agony together in a sack, and walks
with pulling the sack
Sadness and agony
Strong sense of duty and responsibility

<Special Characteristics>
<u>Always hit head at accident or injury</u>
Body is warm
Disorder of water balance
Profuse discharges (yellow, or yellow green)
Yellow green tongue
Indigestion
Symptom like influenza
Hemophilia
Gallstone, problem in liver
Gonorrhoea
Asthma
Diabetes
Warts around eyes, on face or on chest
Oedema (swelling)
Salty phlegm

<Region> Occiput, Liver, Gallbladder, Pancreas, Intestines, Lungs

<Modality>
Worse Dampness, Lie on left side, Injuries (head, spine), Warm and rainy weather, Early morning (4 to 5 am)
Better Fresh air, Dry weather

Natrum-sulph: Case

35 years old   Male
Main complaints: Hepatitis and gout

- Yellow complexion
- Yellowish in white parts in his eyes
- Tends to have diarrhea in summer time
- Always gets hangover after drinking alcohol
- Gets angry easily, and always being irritable
- Suicidal desire
- Warts around eyes has been increased

Nat-sulph 12X x two bottles (approx. 66 pillules)
        Morning, Noon, and Night

Nat-sulph is used for problems in muscles, brains, hyperactivities, gout, joints, and livers. This person tends to hit his/her head. Nat-sulph is the most suitable remedy for a mental disorder, which was started to think to commit suicide since he/she hit a head.
Nat-sulph is also No.1 tissue salts to increase resistance as well as Silica does. When resistance is fallen, athlete's foot, candida, suppuration are easily formed, and Nat-sulph suits those problems.

Silicea
Sil.

<Mind> Mind excels better than physical body, but it gets worse from being overused
Spirited
Nervous temperament and irritable
Picking toys with pins or needles
Difficult to be pleased
Cannot summarise at exams due to thinking too much
Physically weak, but is clever

<Special Characteristics>
Body is very cold
Thirsty
Spurt out foreign bodies in hair, nails, bones, urine, and blood
<u>Weak and malnutrition (lack in absorbency)</u>
Very nervous and small
Stool stops in the middle of the excretion
Offensive perspiration in feet
Vacant and cannot concentrate
Easily gets tired
Headache due to tiredness or too much studying
Children, who like using pins and needles
Bleeds easily
Gangrene and ulcers in bones
Brittle nails
Inflammation and swellings
Healing of injuries on skin is slow
Yellowish and offensive discharges

<Pregnancy> Pain and sluggish in legs
Cracks in nipples
Quality of milk is bad and the baby does not drink it

<Region> Nerves, Glands, Secretion system, Bones, Skin, Ears, Nails, Hair

\<Modality\>
Worse   Chill, Draft, Dampness, Milk, Vaccination, Conventional medicines
Better   Covers a whole body warmly, Hot bath, Rest

Silicea: Case
3 years old Boy
Main complaints: Weak constitution

- Nails are weak and limply
- Small
- Slow growth
- Takes cold easily
- Sensitive to sound, lights, and coldness
- His wounds tend to be suppurated, and heal so slowly
- Profuse sweats in head during sleep
- Sweats in feet during daytime, Sweaty and offensive
- Anyway, he is weak, and takes cold so easily
- When he takes cold, his lymphatic glands are swollen and has to take anti-biotic, but his mother would like to stop this pattern
- He has got hematocele due to the difficult labour (it has become quite small now, though,,,)

Morning	Silica 12X x	one bottle (approx. 33 pillules)
Night 1	Silica 6C x	10 days
Night 2	Silica 200C x	2 days

Silica suits brittle bones, nails and teeth very well, and plays a role of heightening the function of whole tissues in a body.
It suits a constitution, which forms ulcers or pus easily.
Silica is an important remedy for children, who had conventional medicines and vaccinations a lot.
Silica makes walls of vessels to have elasticity. (varices or hemorrhoids)
It lets T cells (immunocyte) activate and makes the body to be strong against infection.

Combination remedies of tissue salts

TS01 (blood) compatible problems: bad quality of blood, anaemia, bad complextion
TS02 (hair) compatible problems: general problems in hair, fallen hair, dull hair (not lustre)
TS03 (nail) compatible problems: general problems in nails
TS04 (stomach) compatible problems: general problems in stomach
TS05 (skin) compatible problems: general problems in skin
TS06 (aging of skin) compatible problems: aging of skin
TS07 (bedsore) compatible problems: bedsore problems
TS08 (migraine) compatible problems: neurosis migraine
TS09 (sciatica) compatible problems: sciatica
TS10 (rheumatism) compatible problems: rheumatism
TS11 (back ache and lumbago) compatible problems: back ache and lumbago
TS12 (muscle pain) compatible problems: muscle pains
TS13 (pain in foot and leg) compatible problems: pain in foot and leg
TS14 (period pain) compatible problems: period pain
TS15 (indigestion (gas)) compatible problems: indigestion, profuse gas emission
TS16 (indigestion (heartburn)) compatible problems: indigestion, heartburn
TS17 (catarrh and sinusitis) compatible problems: catarrh, sinusitis
TS18 (hayfever) compatible problems: hay fever
TS19 (cold) compatible problems: cold in general
TS20 (irritation) compatible problems: irritation, when someone is upset/nervous
TS21 (teeth and bones) compatible problems: general problems in bones and teeth, broken bone, broken teeth, having a tooth extracted. scoliosis, osteoporosis, a period of growth, Eumycetes (fungus such as athlete's foot)
TS22 (milk teeth) compatible problems: teething at infant
Vital salt compatible problems: stagnant of vitality, malnutrition, weak constitution

MATERIA MEDICA OF 12 CELL ACTIVE TISSUE SALTS

Ars-iod
Ars-i.

<Keynotes>
Strong thirst, Gravedo (catarrh in nose) due to hay fever, Asthma, Convulsion in a bronchial tube, Oozing eczema, Acne, Lymphoma, Acne in adolescence

<Mind>
Weak mentality, Headache if overtax his/her brain, Cannot study.
No peace in mind, Always in a hurry.
Always has a complaint somewhere, Never be in a good condition

<Body>
This remedy suits blood and lymph the best. It also suits influenza, hay fever, chronic accessorius catarrh, otitis media, difficulty in hearing, lung cancer, and breast cancer with ulcer.
His/Her hay fever has watery, acid, has burning discharges from nose and sneezes one after another. Due to the hay fever, the condition becomes as if having cold, and has profuse sweat during sleep.
All discharges smell rotten. They are stimulative and turn into a running sore. Although skin is dry, the affected part has oozing yellow discharges, and is difficult to be cured. The discharges cause pain and itch. Scratched part has discharges, being mixed with blood.
It suits to acne and scabies in youth. It is also good for eczema with pus in hair, syphilis constitution, chronic bronchitis and dry cough, which never stop for a long period. The phlegm is yellow green. He/she has hoarse in throat and tendency to become aphonia.
It is also suits to asthma, tuberculosis, and influenza.
It could be called homoeopathic anti-biotic for multiple allergy.

<Modality>
Worse   Tobacco, Current of air

Ars-iod: Case

35 years old   Female
Main complaints: long lasting nasitis and cough

She was suffering from nasitis at all times. Blocked and Runny nose alternate, depending on seasons. She always has sore throat because her nose is blocked during sleep, so she sleeps with opening her mouth. This causes discharges in nose goes into mouth, and she has constant cough, as a result. She cannot spit out phlegm. When she suffers from hay fever, her skin swells red and itch. She used to have otitis media at childhood, and was administered antiseptics into her ears. Her right ear has difficulty in hearing now.

Ars-iod 12X x 2 weeks

Calc-carb
Calc.

<Key notes>
Headache as if it explodes, Lymphadenomatosis, Chronic mucomembranous catarrh,
Thamuria, Enuresis, Children in general, Utterly exhausted condition, Geromorphism

<Special characteristics>
Calc-carb. is one of constitutional remedies, and is normally used in the range of 30C and 200C. However, when we use it in low potency, it can be used as a comfortable remedy to cell tissues.
Calc-carb person tends to gain weight. As their fat metabolism and water metabolism are bad, they accumulate fat and water in their body. Their body is flabby and soft.
Quality of their bones is also bad. Their body is cold, and they have cold sweat in their hands and feet. The sweat smells sour. The constitution is phlegmatic temperament. Babies, who sweat easily and are fat. Babies, whose heads were big, and whose fontanelles were difficult to be closed. Or, people, tend to gain weight, and their skin is whitish or greyish. By taking Calc-carb, these flabby bodies become more firmed up and solid. Their balance of calcium also gets better and the person starts to have much strong bones.
They catch cold easily due to a water related job, such as fishery or farming (esp. rice planting). If we have bad calcium absorption, we have problems in lymph, glands, bones, skin, nerves, an adrenal gland, etc.
Calc-carb suits thyroadenitis, pituitrism, osteomyelitis, and osteoporosis very well.
It suits a person, who feels weakness after climbing mountain, talking and walking, and has a crick or a pulled muscle easily due to carrying a heavy thing. Worse from cold and damp weather. They scare mice.

Calc-carb: Case

8 years old   Girl
Main complaints: She cannot stop coughing. Her hands and feet are smelly.
Her ankles makes noise and are easily sprained

Her birth weight was 3,900g, a big baby. She had adipic eczema and it stayed quite long time. Her skin has elasticity extraordinary and her cheeks stretch so long. She is on the plump side. Her voice gets to be hoarse easily. Guttural voice. She grudges having to work. She hates to climb mountain and gardening. Her lymphonodus is always swollen and has hard lumps. She does not want to watch or hear cruel story. She wants to eat everything as long as it is edible. She ate cat food recently. Her teeth tend to decay easily.

Calc-carb 12X   x   2 weeks

Cuprum-ars
Cupr-ars.

<Key notes>
Shooting pain in head, Tinnitus, Convulsion in muscles, Leg cramps, Whooping cough,
Nephrocolic, Sciatica, Gastrointestinal problems, Diarrhea

<Mind>
Although the person is spiritless, he/she cares trivial things, and is getting to be nervous breakdown. His/her worries never disappear. 'Am I committing a crime?' 'Will I get ill?' 'Will my diarrhea never stop?' etc.

<Body>
Cuprum conforms to nerves, intestines and toxin in a body. Arsenicum conforms to intestines and kidney and low vitalities.
Cuprum-ars conforms to cholera, typhoid, dysentery, colitis, diarrhea, etc. The patient has cold and sodden sweats and intermittent diarrhea, which is as if heavy oil. He/she has violent pain. These cause weakness and his/her legs cramp during walking and the whole body shakes because it cannot hold the weight. It suits to numbness due to encephalopathia with diarrhea, dizziness, and headache. It is similar to Veratrum-alb and Cuprum.
Their kidney gets uremia and diabetes easily. Their urine smells like garlic, and acetone is excreted a lot. Their skin is cold like ice. They tend to have abscesses on face or genitals, which are easily festered.
Once they start to hiccup, it does not stop so easily. All their symptoms, such as stiff shoulder or back, diarrhea, and so on, get worse from moving.

Cuprum-ars: Case

50 years old   Male
Main complaints: He is always in bad condition. Weakness.

Since he drank water in a ditch, he suffers from autotoxemia. He has diarrhea and fever periodically. His body is cold, but he sweats oozy. Sweating does not ameliorate the condition. As he had a suspicion of having malaria in the past, he received a treatment for that. When he has diarrhea, he desires for water, but if he drinks water, the diarrhea gets worse.
His wife ' I can find whether he used toilet or not, because his urine gets so smelly and the colour becomes thick during he has diarrhea and fever.'
The man ' I am suffering from persistent stiff shoulder on left side. My back also aches.'

Cuprum- ars 12X x 1 week   Morning and Night

Hepar-sulph
Hep.

<Key notes>
Infantile seborrheic eczema, Abscess, Worn out, Utterly exhausted condition, Lost weight

<Special Characteristics>
This remedy is made from oyster shell (Calc-carb) and sulphur, which was burnt in fire, and is similar to Calc-sulph. However, during the process of burning, it becomes Hepar-sulph due to the chemical change. Adaptabilities of Hepar-sulph 30C and Hepar-sulph 12X are different. Hepar-sulph 30C conforms to festered condition and leads to its cure. On the other hand, Hepar-sulph12X conforms to a condition, which toxin is accumulated in a body. If we use it for the condition, it works for collecting wastes, forming pus and excreting outside of the body. Consequently, a person, who tends to have eruptions regularly, Hepar-sulph 30C would match. While, a person, who has a festered abscess, and the pus does not come out easily, would suit to Hepar-sulph 12X. When the pus starts to be broken, the wound part stop being decomposed, or the wound part heals much faster.

<Mind>
They are sensitive to stimulants from outside, such as temperature, sound, lights, people's words or attitudes, and atmosphere. It makes them to fall in utterly exhausted condition. If it is hot, they sweat easily, and complain about it. However, their body is so cold and they cannot leave their blanket even it is hot. They feel cold wind goes through their body and get worse from dampness and coldness. When they take cold thing, such as ice cream, they start to cough and cannot stop it because the coldness stimulates them. Their discharges from nose or ears, and tonsillitis are festered and smell rotten. Their pain is like piercing and burning. Their stomach is flaccid and hung down. They do not have so much appetite, and start to loose weight. They like stimulants, such as sour things and strong flavours. This remedy suits to symptoms, which are caused by mercury toxicity (increased saliva and perspiration, swollen lymphatic glands, tiredness, easily get angry, etc). It also suits to another heavy metal toxicity. It is very good for problems in liver (stagnation of detoxification).

Hepar-sulph: Case

8 years old Boy
Main complaints: An abscess about 3cm in diameter appeared inside of his thigh. It spread over his body, and looks like burned-out and does not heal easily. His body aches. He hates strongly to be touched and take off clothes. He gets angry and abuses his body.

Calc-sulph 12X x	1 bottle (approx. 33 pillules)	Morning
Hepar-sluph 12X x	2 weeks	Night
Bees wax C	At any time	

Kali-alumina-sulph
Kali-al-s

<Key notes>
A fit of headache and cough, Dizziness, Hectic colic, Tympanum colic, Neuropathy,
Dry mouth, Dry skin

<Special Characteristics>
They tend to have gas in their bowels easily. Even they break wind, another gas comes in and keep breaking wind anytime. Although their stool is loose, it does not come out so easily.
Kali-sulph conforms to liver and plays a role of collagen, which makes beautiful skin. Alumina conforms to dry and rough skin, which does not have moist.
Kali-alumina-sulph would be good for a person, who suffers from a problem in intestines and a problem of skin. If the intestines are not cleaned up, the quality of skin gets worse.
Kali-almina-sulph also conforms to nerves as Zincum does. It is best remedy for a person, having imbalance of intestines due to mental exertion (study too much or overtax his/her brain, anxieties).

Kali-alumina-sulph: Case

65 years old Female

Main complaints: Her lower abdomen is swollen paunchy and has gas movements inside. When she cannot break wind, the swell gets worse and she does not feel comfortable. In winter, she gets static electricity easily, and is afraid of touching a car's door or metals. She keeps putting moisturising cream. Her heels are also cracked and ache.

Kali-alumina-sulph 12X x 2 weeks
Beewax Tu At any time

Kali-ars
Kali-ar.

<Key notes>
Skin disorders (Itchy rash, Ulcerative skin disease), Emaciation (Body emaciation, Nervous debility), Nervous anaemia, Runny diarrhoea (worse from coldness)

<Mind>
Panic tendency, nervousness. They are frightened, being anxiety as if they diedeath from heart attack or thrombosis incurred. They are very frightened with their face stiffened and tight, they won't laugh or smile. That is because they are always having a fearful anxiety for illness.
Depressively down and being confined. They get angry for small things, temperamental, and are difficult to handle with. Those are Kali-ars type of people.

<Body>
This is an important remedy for skin problems and emaciation. It is good for herpes on right side, chronic atopic eczema and rash from measles, also fits for a person who looks like getting aging as an old person with having his/her skin gets hardened and becomes yellowish colour.
It also matches for toxins inside the body and blood impurity, being caused by a long-term use of steroid for psoriasis treatment. He/she tends to have ulcer on his/her toes, which gives sever pain. He/she has no power due to emaciation, being unable to put up his/her body on the bed. Any kind of illness turns into malignantly. This is the type of person who has a cold body with shaking in shivering cold.

<Modality>
Worse　　　　Night (AM 1:00 – 3:00), Legs get cold

Kali-ars: case

28 years old Female
Main complaints: Atopic eczema

She had been suffering from atopic eczema since she was a little and she has used steroid for a while. Heavy pigment composure. The body gets cold but even little raise of body temperature makes her very itchy. Thicker beard as a woman. Worrying, anxiety makes her pulsating on such a small things.

Morning   TS-05   <Skin support> x 1 bottle (approx. 33 pillules)
Night   Kali-ars   12X x 2 weeks

Her body chilliness could be caused by her kept using steroid cream. She has to get her natural body in order to reinstate her natural hormonal balance.

Kali-brom
Kali-br.
<Key notes>
Tranquilizer, Insomnia, Neuralgic sight impediment, Depressiveness, State in excitement, Glands problems (especially Thyroid), Amnesia, Suppurations of itchy skin, Acne, Stimulative inflammation, Warmth (cannot stand for warmth)

<Special Characteristics>
Kali-brom is just like as Kali-phos, which is good for nerves and brain. Kali-phos matches with a state of too much use of brain. Kali-brom matches with problems of brain nerves due to their delusion of being damaged by people. Potassium bromide is being used as a medicine for temper in the conventional medicines. But keep taking Kali-bromide as a material incurs opposite reaction, such as a nervous impediment, inactivation of brain and memory, and anaplasia. Kali-brom. is good for, elderly peoples' brains, dementia to keep repeating same things, forgetting speaking, inactivation of brain and verves of melancholia. Also, it is good for occipital migraines with spasm and paralysis on hands that are incurred simultaneously, sexual excitement, the person who gets epilepsy on doing too much sex. The person who has strong sexual desires but no sexual energy to go with, the remedies for this kind of person is Selenium or Kali-brom. Kali-brom. also has a character of moving hands all the time and not be able to stop it. (Zinc has cramp and moving motion in their legs.) It works for repetitive diarrhoea, and cholera too. Kali-brom. relieves brain stimulation that is caused by rectum, which tends to have diarrhoea. Also good for people, who have ulcerative colitis and always want to evacuate stools. Also this remedy is good for children, who keep sleeping with emaciation from cholera.

<Mind>
Violent emotional undulation causes them cry suddenly. They get angry and are fearful.
Doubtful to people by imagining of being poisoned to or to be abused. They believe that they will be punished by heaven. Their memory is punctuated that they can't remember much of the past but remember vividly about disliked incidents in the past.

Kali-brom: Case

65 years old   Female
Main complaints: Sleeplessness caused by diabetes and themuria.
She has been taking sleeping medicine and stabilizer for a long time.

Her son says, she is a little weak-headed and when she is asked about her past, she doesn't remember most of anything. When I ask her about the centre of her mind she evades the point as saying "so many things happen in a life". Still trying to ask her that, she replies "Why do you ask so many about other people's matters?". She deplores that she can't enjoy the meal, can't have a good relationship with people and her life is meaningless. Following is the 2nd time consultation for her.

<Mother=M> "I'm continuously hearing the song in my ear which I listened to in my young days. You, what did you let me have taken? What are you trying to do to me with chasing my past."
<Yui=Y> "There was a lot of unfortunates happened on you in the past, wasn't it? You did cover up those things, that's why you are attending this situation. The lid of your mind had been taken out. So, let's hang on there to push out of those things."
<M> "I won't take it any more."
<Son> "Mother, let's keep taking it. If you don't take it, you become weaker in head and ended up you don't know who you are."
<M> "I've never ever been given any supports by my husband financially or morally. Bringing up my children, caring mother in law, all I did it myself. When I just got myself ease after all the hard works, my husband who was giving me such a hard time, died. I just wanted him to say the word "Thank you" to me."
<Y> "You have kept thinking about it all the time, haven't you? You are never able to accept that point, aren't you? You got to be sleepless while you couldn't be relaxed in your every day life. Once, you had better make complain and speak loudly of

your bear mind to your husband who is being set in a family alter, who even didn't say the word thank you. Then, you would find many things, which you could appreciate in every day life that will bring you something wonderful. You'd better take one more bottle of Kali-brom. for relaxing your brain nerves."

Kali-iod
Kali-i.

<Key notes>
Arthrophyma, Rheumatism, Sciatica, Chronic infection, Cold red hands, Thyroid problems, High blood pressure, Calcification (Stiffness), Deterioration, Lymphatic tumour

<Mind>
They speak a lot and make meaningless jokes mostly. Frightened by only a little sound and cry for uneasiness. She hits, abuses her husband and her children, gets crossed and becomes short tempered. They cannot sit still at all due to pains and anxiety. They distract themselves with walking around irritatingly. They are not capable to communicate with others in right words. Kali-iod. type of people like outside air and they will not get tired walking around outside.

<Body>
Kali-iod. is a remedy for people who easily get haemorrhage. Their bleeding can't be stopped, and they have a tendency of getting oedema. The oedema is incurred in large joints or joint tissues, and that cause rheumatism and sciatica. The rheumatic pain gets worse at night and in dampness and it has to be removed water by syringe. Even water is removed by syringe, soon again oedema comes back. It is important to take Kali-iod for a long period for those people who need to excrete poisonings, which are in joint tissues and fibrous tissues.
They tend to have thyroid problems, and their throat and their tonsils are tingling with pain.
They don't like to wear tight things around their neck. They often cough and their phlegm contains yellow green coloured bubbles.
Also, this remedy is good for rachitis and rachiocampsis, which are incurred by destruction of bones with permeation through bone tissues, acute rhinitis, tumour, condyloma, lymphatic tumour, and cancer.
There are Tubercular miasm and Syphilis miasm, considering from symptoms of Kali-iod.
In fact, Kali-iod is used in conformity with Tuberculosis and Syphilis.

Kali – iod.: Case

45 years old   Female
Main complaints: Rheumatism. Pain and swelling on her knees and her wrists.

Water was removed by syringe for 10 times. Rheumatism gets worse when dampness is high. Coughings and phlegms don't stop. Having rhinitis a whole year. Heavy tinnitus with light dizziness.
There are two large myomas but they are left being not touched. The genital discharge has bad smell, and a lot of quantity.
Anxiety and strong obsession, always being irritated.
She had worked for a job for 10 years, but nobody approved her as much as she expected, and relationships with others at work wasn't so good. She has been angry, and has been worrying agonisingly. She became rheumatism and gave up the job in the end.

Kali-iod. 12X x 2 weeks

Lithium-mur
Lith-m.

<Key notes>
Headaches (>Eating), Hypochondria, Neurolysis, Chronic synarthrophysis (Joint stiffness), Rheumatism, Intraintestinal gas, Deterioration, Gout

<Mind>
They don't have even a single hope and very depressive, fed up with living. They think that they are alone and no help is given by anybody. This thought makes them tend to think there is nothing interesting thing in their life. Their basic problem is a relationship with their mother. If their experience, which they received no security from their mother or father, was happened a lot at embryo, at birth, infant days, it brings them up to be an adult, who has no hope to look up in solidarity and has no help from anybody. That is why Lithium-mur is a remedy for people, who easily go down and become depressive.
Lithium is being used for anti-depression and tranquilizer. The harmful effects of these medicines are tinnitus, feeling face heavy and distrait, and getting dizzy.
Lithium-mur suits for medicinal poisonings. The body starts to act positively discharging the medicinal poisonings by taking Lithium-mur.

<Body>
Hungry stomach gives headaches and feel his/her head has become bigger. The headache stays until they eat something. But too much eat brings heartburn. Rheumatism pain gets worse as if being stung when taking a hot bath. There is numbness on the tongue and speaks as a tongue-tied. A body suffers from emaciation, tinnitus, continuous dizziness, always being accompanied with discomforting nausea. The skin is dried up roughly as Almina, itchiness all the time, gets raw in scratch. It particularly appears on hands, head, and cheeks. Lithium-mur suits for gout, rheumatic pains, strain of nerves.

Lithium-mur: Case

45 years old   Male
Main complaints: Depression

He feels his body heavy. He feels that he cannot hold his body and move. When he stays posing a position that stops blood circulation, he gets numbness and to be paralyzed.
The sight of view is as if it is waving, so he feels he might fall down. Lying on left side causes tinnitus with hollow sound. He cannot recognize taste. He gets mouth ulcers easily.
Sometimes, squeezing pain felt on his heart.
He lost a love around 22 years old, when he just started working. His mother had passed away, and he's been carrying his life in solitude. He took sleeping pills and anti-depressive medicine for 2 years at that time. It is hard to think if he has been living a good life until now.
Everything was so hard in his life and his mother had gone past without having a proper talk. He really wanted to have behaved like a pampered child. His body can't be relaxed as he subconsciously prepares a situation of anything bad again. He worries instantly, tends to be depressive, and dislikes to go out to see people.

Lithium-mur   12X x 2 weeks

Manganum-sulph
Mang-s.

<Key notes>
Nervous break down, Muscle shake, Circulation impediment, State of exhaustion, Declining of memorisation, Nervous breakdown, Anaemia, Deterioration, Lacking of iron

<Special Characteristics>
It plays a role of promoting iron absorption. Iron is absorbed in intestine to produce haemoglobin, which carries oxygen in blood. As a reason why there is lacking of this element, a poor activity of intestines could be listed.

Mangan-sulph is good for people, who tend to have a lack of digestive absorption digestion by diarrhoea, which is caused by an abnormal biliation of digestive enzymes secretion from large and small intestines. Their stools are golden brown coloured, viscous, and smell like a rotten egg.

It also causes a problem on a digestion, having too little biliation of cholecyst.

Mangan-sulph works for controlling bile that reduces it for people, who have it too much, and increases it for people, who are short of it. It is also good for liver, which is deeply related to the cholecyst. It gives activation to liver.

It works for pain on sweet teeth. Also, is good for problems of shoulders, chest, jaw, gastroenteritis, bile disturbance, liver, and pancreas.

In mental sphere, there is no endurance for anything. They easily get angry for trivial things.

For example, he/she gets angry for children, who make loud voice. They can't go along with others.

Manganum-sulph: Case

18 years old   Female

Dizziness and loss of appetite, diarrhoea in period. Any small movement flushes her face red. She had been having diarrhoea for a while when she was a baby. Easily gets bruises. Her whole body is aching. She walks jerkily and falls easily.

Morning   Purifying blood <support>   x 1 bottle (approx. 33 pillules)
Night   Mangan-sulph   12X x 2 weeks

Natrum-bicarb
Nat-bic.

<Key notes>
Deep coloured blood, Very thick blood, Excess of uric acid in blood, Inactive metabolism (discharging of wastes is not working sufficiently), Adiposis, Rheumatism, Thirst, Hates meat and fat, Unacceptable for vegetables and milk, Night sweat, Frigidity

<Special Characteristics>
Nat-carb is contained in pancreas and is effective to pancreatitis.
It prevents oxidization inside the body with accelerating cells in alkalescence, and promotes metabolism and excretion of internal wastes. It is good for inflammation that is caused by stomach acid, urinal acid, acid in the esophagus, also for stomach ulcer and intestinal ulcer (enterelcosis). Taking Nat-phos and Nat-bicarb together neutralize internal activated oxygen to make the constitution be anti-cancerous. Nat-bicarb is effective for as follows: Belching a lot, Dizziness, Tinnitus, Nausea, Short of oxygen to get carbon dioxide poisoning, Symptoms of Mountain Sickness, When heat of the body is retained inside. It is also good for lots of moist retained inside the body, and having dropsy.

Natrum-bicarb : Case

40 years old   Female
Main complaints: Heartburn and indigestion.

No concentration and being forgetfulness. Although she's got a weak digestive system. She likes sweets, bread, butter and coffee. She gets diarrhea and retains gas when she eats those. She likes to drink coffee, which refreshes her from muddled head and it helps for urination. (Nat-bicarb is lacked by drinking coffee or eating snacks quite often).
She suffers from athlete foot, and sometimes gets vaginitis. She is always carrying a sunshade in summer, as she is exhausted when exposed in sunlight.
Nat-bicarb   12X x 1 bottle (33 pillules)   Morning and Night
2 weeks interval
Nat-carb   <Constitutional treatment>   200C x 2 days

2nd Interview
I didn't get on well with my family, but I made a phone call to my father to talk about my childhoods. That was the first time event. I found out that I wanted to be loved by my father.

Nat-carb   10M x 2 days

Zincum-mur
Zinc-m.

<Key notes>
Headaches and oppression at the root of nose, Nervous Breakdown (Prostration), Insomnia,
Memory decline, Hypochondria, Over sensitive to noise, Heat in sole,
Skin itchiness,
Deterioration, Menstrual pain

<Special Characteristics>
Zincum-muriaticum used to be used for a lot as a disinfectant / an antiseptic and sterilizer.
Zincum-mur stimulates metabolism to calm nervous system, and settles menstrual pain with scarce discharge of blood. Even they don't have any appetite, they have a desire to take stimulants or herbs, which affect stomach and intestines badly. They vomit most of everything they eat except for hot milk. One of their character is unrecognizable of smells and tastes. This remedy speeds up curing wounds. When this remedy is taken, we can avoid corruption and can let wounds to close quicker. Zincum-mur is good for people, who are skinny and pale coloured face, having nausea and vomit. This is a remedy for right side extremities paralysis, tics on face, chorea. It also fits for crump, diphtheria, dysentery, anemia and dropsy, getting skinny, although they eat properly. It is good for typhus, injuries, hiccups, which won't stop, constipation, and brain concussion.

Zincum-mur : Case

45 years old   Female

She wants to eat green leaves, especially only lemonberm. She feels nausea if she eats other things. Inside of her mouth is numb and she has no taste at all. She has very heavy period pain with mastitis. Her right side leg is felt heavy and powerless. Twitching under eyes. She collapses with anaemia after taking a bath. She often forgets what she was doing. She cannot remember events. Dropsy and swelling of breasts are eased when period starts.

Zincum-mur   12C x 1 week

MATERIA MEDICA OF OTHER ESSENTIAL TRACE ELEMENTS

Borax
Bor.

<Mind>
Borax children are anxious and fearful, as they are sensitive, and they are difficult to be brought up. Even ring tones of telephone or mother's sneezing frighten them to wake up at night. They scream in sleep, and cry without any reasons. They never get off from their mother, being frightened to strangers and new environment. Can't get down from height, call their mother for help with crying loudly. They can't ride on jet coaster, and can't use elevator even after they are grown up. They can't say 'NO' as they are afraid of people, so they become introverted little by little. Borax people are not grounded. Their personality is not formed firmly, and put them into confusion, and let them be unable to decide or judge. They are always seeking for a guardian or a person in charge for them, having a tendency of becoming dependant. They can't know themselves and they do not have self-confidence.

There are reasons to be thought what draws them into those characters are. They could have kept being ignored, abused, or in tension. There might have been absence of parents or guardians, addiction, and hard labour at birth. Or they didn't drink mother's milk, had lack of relationship with their mother, etc. Those cause them to loose their own self and they become to have a multiple personality.

<Body>
Conjunctivitis.
Trichiasis.
Looking down to get dizzy.
Feel floating in the air when get on a car.
Their hair tend to shrink.
Blocked nose, alternating right side and left side.
Can't drink mother's milk with stomatitis (Aphthosis).
Candida (when mother has Candida, it is recommended that mother needs to take a remedy for letting baby takes it through her breast feed.).
Pasty vaginal discharge.
Children's vaginitis and nappy rash.

Screaming for pain on stools and urination but become cheerful after.
Almost no urination in daytimes but very often at night.
Getting blisters on a face easily.
Mother's milk tastes bad then baby doesn't drink, or if a baby drinks it, it gives baby diarrhoea, abdominal pain or stomatitis.
Herpes.
This causes increases of salivary, osteoporosis, stripping nails, and herpes.

<Region>
Mouth, Nerves, Mucus membranes, Skin, Kidney, Bladder

<Modality>
Worse   Movement of dropping, Sudden sound, Cold, Getting wet, Diarrhoea with fruits,
        Salty, Sour foods, Anxiety, Worry, No cares
Better   1pm, Oppression, Under care

Borax :Case

35 years old mother and 2 years old child
Main complaints: The mother who can't bring up her child and the child who are always eating.

As she had such a bad experience of abusiveness from her mother, she wanted to leave her home in her early age. Luckily she met her gentle husband young. However, after she had a baby she's got very heavy depression and it puts her with no confidence for bringing her child up. She doesn't know how to give a care to the child. When she feels good she pampers the child as a kitten but when she is angry, she leaves the child behind and never touches. This child keeps quiet while being fed with, so this mother keeps feeding snacks all the time. But salty things seem to irritate inside the children's mouth, so he puts a hand in the mouth and repeats crying and eating. When something to eat is disappeared, cries again. He has a pot belly. He has atopic eczema, which covers his face in bright red. Mother doesn't like to be looked at. Trichiasis. Her hair is too rough to be able to be combed. In a first year, she fed her milk but she disliked to be sucked. She has a fear of her emotion, as if she attempts to kill the child one day. She wonders if she has a double personality.

Mother
1. Borax   <Support>   12X x 2 weeks
2. Borax   <Constitutional Treatment>   200C x 2 days
   2 weeks interval
3. Anacardium   <Double personality>   200C x 2 days

Child
1. Antim-crud   <Keep eating due to lack of love>   200C x 2 days
   2 weeks interval
2. Borax   <Constitutional Treatment>   200C x 2 days

Chromium
Chrom.

<Mind>
Dislikes to be humiliated. Does not want to be looked incapable. Challenges things.
Struggle. Gaining carefully step by step. Worries small thing and blames him/herself. Keeps up appearance. Shows his/her capability of a job where nobody there. Wants to prove own ability but won't show true self because of being shy. Patience, could be called cohesive. Perseverance.

<Body>
Stops inflammations.
Smelly sweat and secretions.
Bleeding from haemorrhoid.
Diphtheria.
Throat pain.
Herpes.
Rheumatism in big joints such as a neck, shoulders, and knees.
Diabetes and gout.
Tuberculosis.
Symptoms start acutely and cease suddenly

<Modality>
Worse   5am, Wheat, Sugar
Better   When he/she is admitted, When he/she accomplished, When nobody is watching

Chromium : Case

21 years old   Male (on writing a graduation thesis)

He is being evaluated excellent at the university, and he is very much fulfilling the expectations from his teachers and parents. He looks brilliantly, being a neat and tidy smart youngman. He has a joint pain especially on his neck as he is always looking down to do writings. Bleeding from haemorrhoid gets worse if he sits for long hours. Sweat and snivel smell badly. He can concentrate on studying the best after midnight till early morning. When somebody is with him, he cannot study. He likes sweets.

Morning   Cobaltum   12C x 1 week
Night   Chromium   12C x 1 week

Chromium raises saccharo metabolism to produce energy for hard using of brain to prepare exam or make a job plan. Cobaltum raises immunity and cleans blood, so circulation can reach the whole body, and brain can be activated.

Cobaltum
Cob.

<Mind>
They have an impatient mind and worry about bits and pieces yet doing things over and over again. Being anxious for future in loosing confidence even he/she has achievable abilities.
Preparing things firmly to avoid making mistakes.
Does not want to talk about self. Does not want to be stared at.
(As he/she is convinced that he/she has lacked something.)
Does not want to make any mistakes as he/she wants to achieve perfectly. Thinking themselves as too powerless.
Having a sense of guilt, getting nervous when a policeman approaches him/her (mind of being criminal).
Dream of; Trying to go further ahead but can't. Can't make it on time. Being disturbed by people. An attempt won't be succeeded.

?Nux-vomica fits for stress of people today. However, other element remedies, Cobaltum, Zincum, Osmium, Rhodium, Iridium will match better to stresses, which arise from much deep reasons.

<Body>
Lack of blood solidification. Malignant anaemia. Impotent. Ejaculation without erection. Tearful in open air. Aversion to sours. Aggravate at cold and damp places.
Aggravate at 5 am. Resisting power goes down. Lower back pain.
Weak knees. Crack lips. Cleft palate. Swollen tongue. Lung, tongue, throat, esophagus
Cancer. Growth impediment. Spondyloschisis.

<Modality>
Worse   Morning, Travel on the car, Train
Better Early afternoon to evening, Belch

Cobaltum: Case

17 years old   A high school student, preparing for university entrance exam.
Main complaints: Panic attack
He blames himself as being a loose and hopeless even he is studying more than 5 hours after school. He was so nervous at pre-exam held last time, his head became empty as everything vanished in white and he could not remember anything at all. He is now giving up university exams after this has happened. He drives his brain too hard, and this causesmore sleeplessness. He gets up 5 o'clock in the morning even how late he goes to sleep.
He has no refreshed feelings after sleep. Mosquito bites were infected for a long while andhave left him scars. He has nosebleed, which is hard to stop. He starts shaking and stuttering when he gets nervous.

Cobaltum   12C x 1 week   Morning and Night

2-3 days after he started to take this remedy, he suddenly said, "I go to bed" around 10 pm.
He was left asleep as he was sleeping so deeply next morning. Usually he gets panic and complains why nobody woke him up, but he just changed his clothes calmly and went to school. His style of studying at night has been changed into starting straight after school,
and he now goes to bed around 11pm and gets up at 5:00 in the morning to study again.
He is doing things in his own pace without becoming panicked now-a-days. He seems not to concern about the exam so much. His timidly behaviour has also been improved.

Next remedy is Zincum (Zinc). This is good for people, who drive their brain so hard and have a crowded head.

Germanium
Germ.

<Mind>
They are just like as a bureaucrats type of people, working busy everyday but they don't want to take any responsibilities more than they are committing now. Their intension is to keep rules and to maintain the repetition of everyday routine, living like a robot. Even if they are filled with emptiness and possessed with spiritless, they try to disguise everything is in right order and goes well. They are the type of people, who try to avoid responsibility given, and intentionally push it over to other people. They are terrified of being removed their mask, which they cover up themselves. They think that the best way to avoid failures is to keep holding the present situation, and try to do things as the formality. Germanium fits for; a precise people who like to repeat same things everyday, have no romance, have no hopes, have no dreams, and are ostensible with a mere shadow of themselves. They have dreams, such as making wasted effort, missing bus, leaving their belongings behind, being chased by police.

<Body>
They have a paralysis feeling, shaking legs, may become dysphasia and dyslexia. The reason why those are incurred should be due to problems on their cerebellum and mind.
Germanium is for; cancer, malaria, smarting on throat with lot of mucus, tuberculosis, bronchitis, liver and kidney damages, high blood pressure, anaemia, diabetes, arthritis, skin diseases with nodules, and so on.

<Modality>
Worse   Cold, Mist, 5am

Germanium :Case

38 years old   Male
Main complaints: Pain on his knee joints. Epithelial crescent is worn out. He had a surgical operation for empyema at his young age.
His nose gets blocked easily.
He is working in town office. There is no expression on his face. He doesn't even smile when I told a joke. Prescribed Arg-met, Stannum, Rhus-tox, Kali-bich, Ledum, but the response was not so much than being expected.

<Yui>   "What is your future dream?'
<Patient> "I bought a home, though I keep working as a civil servant for the time being to pay my mortgage. I'll think my dream after my retirement."

His motto is to avoid having any frictions with others and keeps himself quiet. He likes to watch sports on TV, play PC, and read books. His children and wife are troublesome. His wife is working at the same place with leaving their children at care. They have been working at the same office for a long time. As he only felt she is acceptable, he married her. There is not much emotion of loving her.

Germanium   12X x 1 week   Morning and Night

<Wife> "He is now looking back his family. He had quarrel with his colleague. I think that the old systems in this office should be changed a bit some how."

Molybdenium
Moly.

<Mind>
They want everything to be perfect. Dreaming of falling. Fear of high place. Challenge by his/her own (Spirit of challenge). Proving their own opinions. They make a thing in action, but worrying it might be failed. They have a strong feeling of insult on a failure, and can't leave from that idea for a long time.

<Body>
Sclerose en plaques. Creaks when turn the neck. Muscle tense. Stiffness. Arms pains. Shaking of hands.
The pain from the bottom of the eyes, neck tendons upon headache that incurs eyes blurred and double vision.
Getting to see word characters smaller, and shaking.
Headaches cause vomits.
Disability of hearing is incurred suddenly.
Hissing sound in the ears.
The skin gets dries and crumbly scraped off.
The skin gets itchiness without having any problems such as rashes. White patches.
Genital problems. Impotent. Prostate gland problems. Ovarian cancer. Thamuria. Orchitis.
Molybudenium is good for people, who get easily tired in general, and who are in tendency of overweight with hypothyroidism. This remedy fits for adrenal gland and becomes its energy source.

<Modality>
Worse   Dampness, Coldness, Fatty food
Better   Open air, Cold water, Yawning

Molybdenium : Case

33 years old   Female (Nurse)
Main complaints: Myodesopsia, deafness.

All these symptoms started, when I got a new job. Getting fat and tired. Sleepy. Migraine starts when I get tired. I am a type of person who accomplishes various tasks in silence. I think that I'm underestimated at my work. Weak stomach. It gets worse with sour things. I feel dizzy when I am tired and fuzzy-headed, then I can't think anything. Just like run out ofenergy. Easily get hoarseness with a lot of phlegm.

Molybden   12C x 1 week   Morning and Night

I have been energized, been able to accomplish more tasks, become working as a man at work. I recalled myself working like this before, when I was young.

<Patient> "I have to save my energy a little bit, otherwise I will burn out again. My character is just like that. I blame for myself that I must be neat and tidy.
<Yui>   'That points are likely to be Molybden. It is hard to do things perfectly. Please relax and go slowly and you can cut corners a bit.

Niccolum
Nicc.

<Mind>
They believe that they are standing on the summit to put everyone under their control. They control themselves, as they believe that they should not have any argument or disharmony with others. They are relatively punctilious people, thinking they must not jealous to people, must not be gloomy in front of people, must not show unpleasantness, should not be interested in sex, and so on.
They think that they are much in noble-minded than other people. People who can suppress their emotions in control are Niccolum. They act well-balanced mature person as a adult, but those angers, inconsistency, and fears are raised inside them.
Their relationships with others are only on surface. Deep understanding in conversationcannot be made. In dream, they are distressed, as they cannot solve exam questions. Truly, they are almost panicking on the day of the real exam.

<Body>
Periodical headache. Successive dry coughs. It gets better to bend forward when coughing.
It is getting worse at night. There is a sour throat and hoarseness (the throat pain goes up to ears.). Cancer. Paralysis. Giddiness. Lots of hiccups. Inflammation on gums. Anaemia.
Liver, pancreas problems. Diabetes. Diarrhoea. Tendency of miscarriage. It continues a bad condition on stomach and being satisfied with small food.

<Modality>
Worse   Motion, Throat gets sore if they talk or yawn, After midnight, Oppression,
        It gets worse periodically
Better Open air, Evening, Cold things, After meal

Niccolum : Case
45 year old   Male (Managing director / Second generation)
Main complaints: The weak teeth, which chip from the base.
There are many fillings, as if robot's teeth (Silver teeth).
Whole body skin are itchy. Especially neck and hair.
His elbows, his wrists, and his fingers ache.
Eating only a little. He gets coughing easily, followed by sticky phlegm. He often has bad breath.

It is hard to make a speech in front of people because of my nervousness, but my job requires me to speak in front of people, so I get used to doing it. I establish communications well with other people, but only on surface relationship, because, if I find out a somebody's problem and get involved with it, it will be troublesome for me. I don't show my emotions much. My mother was not good at establishing relationships and she was always in trouble with others, that is why I don't want to make any frictions with people.
I am very careful on this point. I don't want to have any children, nor particular woman as my wife. I can't have any intensions to form a family. I'm still single. I don't like to hear deep emotional talks. I can't see myself clearly. I want everything to set in peace and keep myself into a peace-at-any price principle.

Niccolum people have ideas that they want to be staying in peace, 'it's OK for myself as I am, I don't need to change anything'. Niccolum is good for people, who think that they are always calm and wonder why other people fight all the time. Niccolum denies maturity as human beings at this present times. Less understanding of self and other people's emotions than Niccolum, is Plumbom.

Niccolum   12X x 1 week   Morning and Night

Osmium
Osm.

This remedy is good for people, who must accomplish any matter with their perseverance.
It is in peak of stress and pressure but Osmium people surely get over it with their patience and perseverance. There must have an Osmium organiser to build up an organisation and a basic. They try to make an effort to help people in trouble and the weaks. They are willing to do heavily pressurised job under heavy responsibilities. They have an active power, so they look like a dictatorial, and the oppositions and lazy people dislike them.

<Mind>
Short-tempered, Restless, Intellectual, Stubborn, Want to help

<Body>
Over sensitive.
Restless.
Sleeplessness, no refreshes after sleep, sleep only for short time.
Numbness on extremities in wake up.
Muscle contraction and stiffness
Parkinson's disease
Multiple sclerosis
Cancer
Eye problems, Glaucoma, Eye pressure, Sight impediment
Heart and vessel problems, High blood pressure, Thrombosis, Cerebral hemorrhage, Anaemia.
Gassy stomach, Wind is very badly smell.
Metrorrhagia, Getting worse on giving birth, pregnancy, menstruation.

<Modality>

Worse   Dampness, Sweating, Sleepiness, Clouded sky, Oppression,
         6 - 9pm, Resting, Bringing up children, House work
Better   Open air, Working, Eating, Pressure, Walking

Osmium : Case

45 years old   Female (Centre manager of Child counselling centre)

My eye pressure on right side is high, and I have pain in the bottom of eye. Blood pressure is high. The body is jerk and stiff. Sleeplessness. It is difficult to go sleep by thinking bits and pieces about job for next day. There is a pain on the joint of right side shin. It's swollen.
Can't sit upright. Weak stomach and intestines and easily gets gassy stomach. Much acid in my stomach. Once start coughing that won't stop. I don't have any time to amuse myself because there are so many things to do. My husband died with leaving two sons, one is at high school and the other is at university. I must work for school fees and food. I get up early every morning for washing and making breakfast and lunch for my son in high school.
I leave home at 8 o'clock in the morning and come back at around 6 in the evening to cook dinner. I have worked very hard. I could not help stopping the job because I was a single parent to bring the two sons up. I became a centre manager finally upon my nature of strong responsibility and I could work with no sleep. It's almost 10 years since engaged this job. It is getting hard to manage my body these days. To be honest, I don't like housework and I didn't like bringing up children. But I have to look after them, who are my own children, and that are upon my responsibility.

Osmium 12X x 1 week   Morning and Night

My body has started to be able to have deep sleep 1 week after I started to take the remedy.
I was working restlessly but have started to be able to manage the job efficiently. I became gentle to my children. I used to be angry and shout to them if they didn't do what I said. My son in university is now often coming back home. My awakening awfulness has been taken away, maybe because my blood pressure went down.

Osmium is good for people, who use their spirit harshly under the stress everyday, always keep them busy, and walk just looks like as their will drags their body.

Rubidium-mur
Rubid-m.

<Mind>
They are impulsive and cannot have careful consideration. Going straight to the aim and don't be bothered by evaluations done by other people. Ideas are sprang out, and they often make mistakes by doing it impulsively. When they failed, they become negative without looking back the reason why they failed, then become to be depressive and negligence. They are even livelier if they are creative, but got to be depressive that become to be self-denial and avoid seeing people. But most of Rubidium person is creative, warm hearted, open minded, and easily interchangeable to others, people are fond of him and he makes many friends. Jean Sholton said "Rubidium is just like as a Boris Becker who won the Wimbledon at the age of 17. He was as a new comer, challenging to those first class players without having any fears. He never thought about a win or loose, just played good games." They sometimes look like haughty but they are just doing what they want to do. Manic state and depressive state come by turns, and they have volatile emotions as crying and laughing. They have a delusion, which many coloured balloons and balls are floating in the air.

<Body>
Easily get visual impediment and eye inflammation.
Stuttering.
Voice won't come out.
Hoarseness.
Liver problems.
Lang problems.
Neck problems.
Stiff joints.
Aching arms.
Weak muscles.
Sleeplessness.
Turning over a lot in sleep.
Jean says, "Rubidium tends to be accumulated in a brain tumour, it's easily observed by scan. Rubidium is able to absorb oxygen immediately

in the process of its oxidization, and I think that it rises the absorption of oxygen in the body."

<Modality>

Worse   5am, September, Before menses, Disciplines, Smell of bay leaf, Clouded dull weather
Better   Outside

Rubidium-mur: Case

Female
I want myself to be special. I have been hoping to obtain a thing, which no one has got, and it became to real at last. This is a fun I am devoting myself into it without looking back my family. I don't want to change this lifestyle even my husband and my son make complains about me. I might be divorced for holding this situation. But I don't want to go back to old myself (there was empty with no soul inside of me).

<Yui> "Both of your minds shall mutually be settled. You shall not determine to take one of either. There is a remedy for comply with."

Rubidium 9C x 10 days

Selenium
Sel.

<Mind>
Extremely sorrow. Being attached by desperation. No enjoyment. Forgetful.
No concentration and unable to think. Not a diplomatic. Sensitive to sound, and voice of People's talking. Often erotic ideas come up in mind, but impotent disturbs to do sex.

<Body>
Hairs come off easily. Hairs are greasy and sticky.
Totally exhausted. No energy.
Thamuria and dropping urine. Prostatitis.
Impotent. Watery and runny semen.
Acne and eruptions are infectious.
Easily get drunk.
Detoxication of mercury.
The heart pulsates when lying down.
Abdominal pulsation(bounce when put a hand onto the abdomen).
Sleeplessness. Being bothered with erotic dreams.
Chronic laryngitis, using voice gets hoarseness easily.
Especially this remedy is used for exhaustion after recent illness.
Gets worse in sunlight, and exhausted in hot weather.
People who have troubles in liver and veins.
Gets worse from tea and alcohol.

<Modality>

Worse   Sleeplessness, Wake up, Ejaculation, Exertion of the brain and the body, Draft, Sun, Hot weather
Better Cool air after sunset, Cold water

Selinium : Case

38 years old   Male (Upper listed farm salaried man)
Main complaints: M.E. Chronic fatigue syndrome

Always being languid (tired), going to work unwillingly. Nobody in my office understands me and they say I am lazy. I don't want to meet people. Can't be diplomatic. Want to go home as soon as possible and lay down. Sweat a lot during sleep. I have nightmares and dream of hard labour. Lacking of sleep makes more tired then sleep over 10 hours.
I have been working very hard before I became like this, I have been socialised, and I had had a lot of alcohol drinks, cigarettes, and coffee. I like sports. I was enjoying yacht. Giddiness and tiredness are worse when I am exposed to sunlight, so I wear hat and sun-glasses now-a-days. I'm enchanted by moon. Being afflicted with suicide sometimes. I tear for life, which is very boring and meaningless.
Being depressed. He looks older than his actual age, and has thin hair.

<Yui=Y> "When did you become like this state?"
<Patient=P> "I've been so tired since 2 years ago. No energy left to achieve anything."
<Y>   "Anything happened at that time?"
<P>   "My colleague and I were competing for one position, and I've got it. It's started since then."
<Y>   "You exerted yourself very hard, didn't you?"
<P>   "Yes. I've been staying with my superior until late at work for getting to become his favourite. But I didn't like him in humanly. Life with my wife also became ruined by coming back home late at night."
<Y>   "Please eat with chewing well those foods, which contains full of vitamin E, such as alfalfa, bean sprouts, grated yam, corn oil. Vitamin E is a source of energy and vitality. Selenium is working for the mercury accumulated in the body. Kali-phos is good for a nervous irritation from exhaustion and over tiredness."

Stannum
Stann.

<Mind>
Feel going down. Depressed. Do not want to meet people.
They care about what other people think about them.
Anxiety. The bad memories in a past, and they are recalled.
Dislike to go to public. Being despised and treated insultingly.
No praises given by the people.
Feeling of abandoned, that is why becoming sympathetic to the people who are in the same situation. They are sensitive to discrimination and they like to have argument on that matter. They persist in their past glory, just like as Bothers.
Turn away the core subject, very good at making a beautiful episode.
Keen on getting a free ride at the expense of another, but prefer to take no responsibility.
Get angry easily. Vengeances. Cynic and sarcastic. Nasty.
Their fears are; Human, Poverty, Being looked down by people, High place, Future.

<Body>
Wrists and hands are swollen and paralysed. Legs get numb easily when they sit erect with their legs folded under them. All illnesses get worse little by little.
Pale face. Arthritis and rheumatisms.
Lung troubles (Asthma, Bronchitis, Lung cancer, Pulmonary fibrosis) causes worn out and speechless. Menstrual cycle is early and quantity is large.
Want to bend down because of period pain.
Hysteroptosis. Gastroptosis. Meniere's disease. White spots on the face.

<Modality>
Worse   When using voice, Coldness(Chilliness), 10am, When they go stairs up and down
Better   Open air, Pressure, Cough with discharging phlegm

Stannum: Case

63 years old   Male   Carpenter

When I catch cold, the cough gets worse and won't stop. That causes me to be unable to have meals and loose weight. Feel disgust by my sticky phlegm and the metal taste. I have got painful joints as well as wrists, ankles, and neck. I cannot walk with aching joints especially when having coughs. It is getting hard for me to make motions little by little. Used to be a master carpenter, but leave it to my son now. "Young people now-a-days are hopeless", this thought is just coming up in mind. My son doesn't like me to put a word in his way, and we start arguing straight away. I entered elderly club and became the chair, because I was the youngest and can be active in the club. Every time I find elderly people are despised from listening to their stories, I get angry. As I have experienced the war in my childhood, I might not be able to be relaxed. Stiff body. I am a straight person. My spirit is also hard.

Stannum 12X x 1 week   Morning and Night

It was surprised because my long-term spasmodic coughs have stopped.
I could not walk with aching joints of knees and neck, but all these pains and aches are much less and feel ease in the morning. I have been so impatient for many things to my son, but now I am trying to leave whole responsibility on him because he is exerting himself. Less argument. I'm continuing to stay the chair of the elderly club. I'm not responding so harshly like before.

There was a child's case. He was a captain of baseball team. He started to catch cold easily straight after he left the position, and he had difficulties in his emotions. Stannum worked very well for this boy. Stannum is just conformity with his mind that he could not leave his glory in his past and felt his value might fade little by little.

Storntium-carb
Stront-c.

<Mind>
No concentration. Temperamental. Depression. Anxiety for being criticized. Getting to avoid expressing themselves and obedient (Cinderella syndrome). They don't think they are talented. They are sensitive to beautiful things and arts. Keep silence.
They are shy and won't solve a matter.

<Body>
Bad blood circulation after a surgical operation, and violent shooting pains.
Illness caused by loosing blood (hemorrhage).
Breaking ankles. Bone cancer. Medulla disease.
Abdominal swell caused by constipation. Violent pain in anus.
Hard body. Rheumatisms. Cold body.
Glaring. Epilepsy.

<Modality>

Worse   Motion, After accident, After surgical operations, Menopause, Bleeding, Oil, 2 – 3am
Better   Warm bath, Light, Bright weather, Wear many clothes

Strontium-carb: Case

70 years old   Woman (She was brought by her daughter.)

Main complaints: Bone weakness.

Bones are easily broken when she falls down. Easily gets hard ganglions. The bone of right side jaw is raised, looking like as a "Lamp Cheek Old Man" (Japanese children's story / Hanasaka jiisan). Halluxvalgus.
She doesn't speak much. Just nodding to her daughter's saying.
She is reserved for her subject to be discussed with. She has weak knees and ankles, which often sprain and ache, so she took many X-rays. Her condition is getting to be osteoparosis. Her bones are weak but she inclines to produce unwanted bones and ganglions. She relies on her daughter these days, and is getting older day by day.

Morning Strontium-carb 12X x 2 weeks
Night   Bone support   1 bottle (approx. 33 pillules)

Her symptoms are similar to 'Rhus-tox' (Ivy lacquer).
Plant Ivy Lacquer contains a lot of Strontuim.

Vanadium
Vana.

<Mind>
Prostration. They won't cover up smelly things.
Mind complications (They want to eat but can't eat. wanting to stop over-eating but can't stop.)
There are something, which must be done but cannot do that and leave it to do later. They can't solve things themselves.
They doubt themselves, and behave miserably as 'I might not be able to manage'.
Dependant, easily become addicted (alcohol, coffee, drugs).
The reason why they become like this, the vanadium type of people want to do everything in perfect, but they don't understand that they will fail while they are seeking for the perfect. It is OK as much as they could have done. They cannot allow them to leave it as OK.
They are always afraid timidly for being late on time, missing train, or being failed.

<Body>
It is difficult to take oxygen into the body. The rate of haemoglobin in blood is low (anaemia).
Low activity of phagocyte (which eats macrophage as well as harmful bacteria).
Chronic rheumatism. Cataract. Proteinuria. Diabetes. Abnormal blood sugar rate.
Raising digestion and absorption. Activates of liver and heart functions.
Addisonian disease (getting tired easily by adrenic hormone problems).

This is a remedy for people who are called as a skinny chubby. They are skinny but their fat rate is high. The people like this should bear in mind for not to take things, such as margarine and saccharine. The calorie removed foods create more fat in unnatural manner.
Vanadium is in conformity with the heart and the liver. Those organs are relating to will, and Vanadium person also can be said weak-willed.

<Modality>

Worse   Coldness, No help from others, 7am, Before menses

Vanadium :Case

16 years old   Girl
Main complaints: Over eating. Getting tired. Getting tense. Very changeable emotions.

Once she feels like flying away to heaven, but if any little disappointments happen or any failure feelings, it put her down into heavy depression.
She has a weak volition, giving up so easily. No patience. Easily hurt (particularly on love, friendship, and sibling relation).
On this point   of view, she takes off school at once when she has problems at school. She is worried if she starts to reject attending school.

Vanadium   9C x   10 days

Over-eating is a problem, being caused by psychological problems and by low blood sugar rate as physical problems. Vanadium is good for such type of people.
The girl's mother is a health enthusiast. She ate for her health rather than ate her favourites food while her pregnancy. If this kind of behaviour is kept in a pregnancy, it affects an embryo, and the baby tend to be a child, who have an unbalanced diet.
The important thing is to ask our body and mind what we want to eat, the chosen are usually be nutritiously needed for our body while the mind and the body are being in a healthy state. Feeling of "delicious" accelerates our nutrition.
Vanadium seems to have matched her very well. After she took 1 bottle of the remedies, she now goes to school without taking off school.

MATERIA MEDICA OF BIO ELEMENTS AND ENVIRONMENT ELEMENTS

Alumina
Alum.

<Mind>
They don't know themselves who they are.
The relationship with loved ones (Mother, Children, Husband, Wife, etc.) won't get along.
There is no space for them in their family.
Unable to choose.
They are afraid of knives and blood. If they see it, they are afraid of their own attitude as they can't control themselves what they are going to do. Tempting to suicide.
Delusion of being chased by police, committing a crime.
No concentration. Feel time goes slow. Afraid of falling forward.
Everything won't go well when urged and rushing.
They are the victims of being ill-treated, persuaded to do the job disliked.

<Body>
The whole body is dried up. Their skin, their hair, and their eyes are all dried up.
The skin itchiness causes scratching until bleeding.
Stools don't come out even it's loose. It's hard to sweat and salivate.
No tastes recognised.
Dislike meat and beer.
Like potatoes but get dyspepsia when eat.
Pain in the abdomen (left side).
Easily getting numbness on the legs.
The nails are soft.
Accumulating nose wax easily.
The backbone and the body are stiff.

<Modality>

Worse	Periodically aggravated, Potatoes, Starches, Salt, Junk-food, Warm room or in bed
Better	Evening, Open air, Natural temperature with little dampness, Washing with water

Alumina : Case

13 years old   Boy
Main complaints: Atopic eczema and itchiness. Injury is opened and blood oozes.
Dry skin. His relationship with mother isn't very good.

He laughs loosely even when he is scolded. He can't express what he wants to do. He can't make up his mind straight away. He is bright but he tend to have daydreams all day, being absentminded, so sometimes he can't solve any questions. When I asked him if he gets angry to his mother, who nags him, he said no. She sometimes pats him. When he sees bleeding he starts to be panicked with shock, but he gets easily injured. He has a stool once in three days but always in diarrhoeas. He is slovenly and loose. He is mostly playing computer games. No conversation with his mother. His mother hasn't held him or hugged him before. He is not as lovable as his younger sister. Mother divorced when he was 3 years old, and he was attached to his father very much.

Alumina   12X x 1 week Morning and Night

His skin and his bowel movement got better. He can concentrate on now. He has started to show his emotional feelings of anger and crying. He said that he didn't like her mother for the first time.

<Boy=B> "My little sister possesses mother only for herself. My father isn't here anymore, I don't know whom I can tell about myself."
<Yui=Y> "When you are in trouble, you can tell your mother."
<B>   "Mother is busy for working all the time. If I tell her, I will put her in trouble."
<Y>   "Such a gentle boy you are. But there is a word saying, that's mutual when being in a trouble, or being in a hard time. You should speak to your mother whatever you like, you can be even against her. When you protest now, it's much more natural than being against a parent when you get older. Are you afraid of knives?"
<B>   "Yes, I'm afraid but I want to use it."
       Next remedy is, Alumina-sulph.

Arg-met
Arg-m.

<Mind>
They are always anxious about their health and respond nervously. But they make an effort not to show it to other people. Their pride is high. They want to be recognised and praised by people, and they also like to be in a centre of attention. They like artistic and aesthetic things, and they intend to collect treasures and keep having them. They terrify high places, narrow spaces, crowded places and start to be panicking if they are at such places.
However they won't show it to others like as Arg-nit (Argentum nitricum) type of people.
They look gentle, but their haughtiness and cold-blooded face come out when they get back home. They are in high pride, and humiliation stays inside of them ever.

<Body>
As symptoms of argent poisoning, nervous suffering and paralysis, damaging of cartilage or tumentia, and inflammation of mucus membranes of pharynx are known. Arg-met works very well for those symptoms.
They have a paralysis on general nervous system, and rheumatism on cartilage inflammation. The regions are, on ankle, toes, and fingers. They ache like neuralgia.
It tends to become Parkinson's disease, which has weak concentration and poor memory.
They have a symptom of electricity, running into a head, and could have an epileptic fit sometimes. They keep themselves busy so they might be so exhausted.
When they speak/sing, their voice gets hoarse immediately, and when they write, they get tenosynovitis easily. The symptoms start slowly, increase gradually, and disappear suddenly.
There's a smarting on their larynx and they get hoarseness. Their voice character changes without raising voice loudly.

<Modality>
Worse   Using voice, Emotional tension, Cold dump air
Better   Motion, Coffee, Wearing clothes

Arg-met : Case

30 years old   Male
Main complaints: Swelling of right testicle. Less feeling and trembling on the whole legs. Unable to clear phlegm. Insomnia

Stiff body. Quiet and moderate character. He is working steadily and is contributing to the company. He pretends to be unconcerned for his position in the company, but wants to show his ability at least. He thinks that he is more creative than what people think, but he is not able to show his ability due to being busy for doing other jobs. He has weak teeth and lots of fillings. He has to clear phlegm every morning when he gets up. Grey colour phlegm. The legs are getting thinner and thinner.
"Is my testicle swollen due to having too much masturbation when I was young?", the company cannot be run without my work, but the symptom is getting worse and I'm thinking to leave the job. But, I should not leave when I think about the company's present situation.
Both of his parents have got weak teeth and they have many silver teeth. There has been cartilage problems since his birth.

Morning Arg-met <support>   12X x 2 weeks
Night 1 Arg-met <constitutional treatment> 200C x 2 days

2 weeks interval

Night 2   Calc-fluor <constitutional treatment>   1M x 2 days
          (Cartilage problems, the body stiffness)

Aurum
Aur.

<Mind>
Just like as a company director, who works day and night to accomplish the aims, or a student in prestigious school who studies hard to get enter an established school. They raise their ideal and aims high and they are inclined an ascetic life to go straight to accomplish it. They are very stoic, and worship God. When they find that the aims cannot be achieved, they suddenly jump from a building, or jump into a train. They won't give up things by halfway, so they accomplish their suicide as well.
They just feel that God gives them a punishment and they are so down from the bottom of their bosom, they cannot find a gold shining life in anywhere.
This remedy is good for; Strong sense of responsibility, Strong pride, Trying to be No.1, Keep holding the present position, Unable to laugh and enjoy life, Solitude, and for people who think they are looser in their deep part of mind. They feel qualms of conscience and humble themselves.
Clouded and rainy day depresses them. Perfectionism.

<Body>
There is a severe pain on bones (especially at night) and they want to commit suicide by the pain. Keep pressurise over their heart. They like open air and dislike stuffy atmosphere inside.
Sudden violent fear, anger, self-denial, irritability, and those are uncontrollable but they don't want anybody to know about it.
The orchidocelioplasty in right side. The lustrous, healthy complexion are appeared on the face and that feels like having a full of blood in circulation. There are many disorders on eyes as well as bloodshot, blurred and narrow views, which of all are caused by blood congestion in head, and sleeplessness due to the responsibility taken.

<Modality>
Worse   Emotion, low spirits, Loss of assets, Overstrained nerves, Chillness, Night
Better Cool air, Open air, Cold water, Bathing, Getting warm, Walking, Rest

Aurum : Case

48 years old   Female (Managing director, The Chairman of organization)

There's always a denial feeling at deep in her mind. She is having a sense of guilt and desperation to have come into this world and she cannot prove herself even her job and activities of the organization, which are being well managed and run well. Deep depression, but she tries to let nobody notice it. She has a solitary feeling with making no friends. She only had a mother when she was born and received almost no care from this mother.
Shallow sleep. There is a sharp pain on her hip and knees. Particularly on right side is bad.
It gets worse when she is alone at night. Are my jobs going successful? Will the organization activity survive? She is being pressurised as crushed in the responsibility of keep running the organization.
Serious character. Her pleasure is to travel or enjoy hot spring by herself. She achieved a certain status at young age and earned assets, there she still has 8 gold teeth, which were put 25 years ago. Her teeth were very weak. Her voice is thick as men's. Willed face. She liked to drink but liver problems had been incurred and given it up. A little bit fatty.

1. Aurum <Support>   12X x 1 week   Morning and Night
2. Aurum <Constitutional Treatment> 1M x 2 days

After finished taking remedies, I've been in tears because of the memory of my life in threatening of suicide.

<Yui=Y> "Why did you try to make an attempt at suicide?"
<Patient=P> "When it comes up thinking of, ' I can't achieve my
            target? Is it going wrong?',
            I wonder I   would be ease if I jump now. In the fact that I feel I will be squashed by
            the big responsibility.
<Y>   "How about now?"
<P>   "I normally won't tell people such a thing, I don't want to give in myself. But I got my feel ease when I spoke like this first time."

Bromium
Brom.

<Mind>
They feel as if they are committing a crime and have to run away. They are sacrificed people, who have become criminals or an assailants without noticing it.
Bromium is passionate for everything, and this is the reason for not being able to go along with others and this tends to be exposing raw emotions, which are offensive, and become violent after all. This causes people hurt. They feel guilty on this, and they start to think to escape from this society. Jobless adults are giving up themselves as "I'm such a hopeless guy" with feeling guilty. A sense of guilt could put them in a mental disorder and a sign of this happens are staring at empty sky or toying with fingers, nails endlessly. They are going to have a delusion that God wants to punish them.

<Body>
Heat gives them hoarseness, easy to loose a voice, all colds are started from throat, they get bronchitis and croupy cough, which won't stop, especially get worse at night.
Phlegm doesn't come out and gives suffocation and they breath like through sponge. All these symptoms are incurred by, going in to warm room, day time and exposed in heat.
Going to sea makes all those symptoms better, that is why Bromium is called "Sailors' remedy". It is also good for hardened glands.

<Region>
Larynx, Air passage, Heart, Circulation,
Glands (Parotidean,Thyroid,Ovary,Breast), Left side

<Modality>
Worse   Warm room, Discipline, Over heat, Cool, Air-conditioning in hot weather, Sour foods, After meal
Better   Nose, bleeding, Sea, Horse riding, Shaving beard

Bromium : Case

35 years old   Male

Main complaints: Unable to have sex with wife. No permanent job.

He has changed his job more than 10 times. "I have had known since I was a child that nothing would go right in my life." I've been a naughty boy at primary school, one day money was missing in my classroom then I was somehow timidly looking around that let all in my class have had a suspicion on me. How vexing it was. I wanted to prove my innocence, but I resigned myself to "I'm being regarded with suspicion."
I've been having asthma since I was young. I know that I'd better give up smoking, but I might not live longer. I'm able to have sex with a professional woman. I might not want to take any responsibilities. I have got orchitis before. My present job is, a carrying industrial waste in a lorry. I'm just being thinking how these wastes are going to be. I want to quit this job soon.

<Yui>   "What are you going to do next after you quit this job?"
<Man>   "The land is messed up with pollution and too many people. I can't move freely. It might be good to be a sailor."

Bromium 12X x 2 weeks

Chlorum-aqua
Chlor.

<Mind>
They worry if they become mad. Excited instantly with small things and get angry easily.
Can't remember people's names. Fear of water, sea, waves. Getting depressed if somebody in family members get ill or died, and can't get out of it. Always being in self-pity, they draw people's attention by making themselves sad. Insecure feeling of being left behind, being felt no one will go stay with, being chased into living in hardship and into the solitude. Incubator is a beginning of life, which is left behind and the feeling of no help is given by anybody at that time. That is why this remedy is for people who were in an incubator, too. Also this remedy is good for children who did not have enough protection, attention, care from mother, and for abandoned children. When the children like this get grown up, they want to obtain those all the time but they can't truly be fulfilled, and resulted that their desire becomes too strong to let them loose their love sometimes. Once they lose a love, they cannot get out of a feeling of abandonment. This remedy is good for people, who are sensitive to other people's troubles and sorrows, also for people who disregard themselves, and for people who always care other people.

<Body>
Chlorine dries up a mucus membrane and which causes an oedema. Skin gets rough, dryness, and itchy. It's getting worse by exposed in sun light. Lips will have herpetic blisters (atopic eczema). Sneeze with tingle feeling in a nose when getting up in the morning, watery runny nose won't stop, and there is a smoky feeling inside the nose. There are characteristics pain of mucus membranes in a nose and bloodshot eyes after swim in a pool. Weak in dampness, easily having a cough, this causes hoarseness (asthma) and a tendency of repetition to catch diphtheria and laryngitis. Inside of mouth is dried up all the time and drink water but tap water contains chlorine then to attend vice circulation. Like salt. Dislike meat.

<Modality>

Worse   From midnight to 7am, Lying down (nose will be blocked), Steeps, Water, Pool, Before menses, Damp (Thirsty)
Better   Open air (cough and bronchi, but tearing)

Chlorum-aqua : Case

7 years old   Girl
Main complaints: Swollen thyroid glands and a slight fever.

Her voice is always hoarse and little bit lower as a child. Mother explains that the girl was left cry out when she was a little. Her thyroid glands are always swollen. Every time when she goes to swimming pool, she catches a cold, an otitis media and gets her skin dried and itchy. When mother can't avoid taking her to the office sometimes with having boss's permission to bring her, she tries to draw an attention from all the staff and she is delighted to be called 'Cutie', or 'Good Girl'. When mother gives her a scolding, she is sulky for quite a while. She can't watch melancholic TV programs. She is crying for her life as weepy and hard. She is a little bit of asthmatic.

<Mother> "By the way, can a water purifier remove chlorine in tap water?"
<Yui>   "Not perfectly, I think. Please take this remedy."

Chlorium-aqua 6C x 2 weeks

Cuprum
Cupr.

<Mind>
They want to be staying along with rules. They want to obey the law. They are very square
and strict. They don't take any excuses. They control themselves firmly. Work more than
being needed. Extremities move unconsciously when they are startled.
They hate to be given a word by others and protect themselves from being told.
They get frustrated if people won't keep rules.
They compel people to obey rules even to people, who are ill in bed.

<Body>
Muscle spasms. Bronchial paralysis. Cramps on feet and toes.
Epilepsy. Convulsion with a high fever. Chorea. Encephalitis.
Whooping cough. Cough doesn't stop.
Metallic taste in the mouth.
Anaemia.
When they take liquid, it makes a rattling sound, then it goes down to the stomach.
Curly hair tendency (is caused by disturbance of cupper, which affects the intestinal absorption.
Also this could be caused by mercury.)
Insufficient formation of bones.
Lack of a pigment (hair and skin).

<Modality>
Worse   Fear or be startled from, Sleeplessness, Head and Abdominal
        pain, Immunocompromised due to exertion of the body.
Better Cold drinks.

Cuprum : Case

50 years old   Male
Main complaints: Left side Headache. Muscle spasms on extremities. Rheumatism.

Normally he is a nice gentle man. However, one day he got angry, biting his lips with having a pale face, and he ended up with collapsing. After this happening, he gets a spasm pain in his heart when he gets angry or gets excited.

<Yui=Y>   "Why did you get so angry when you collapsed?"
<Male=M>   "I had a quarrel with my boss. Company rode us hard at economic booming period in 70's and we worked so hard as oxen. They are urging us early redundancy nowadays, we are being pushed over the corner and handled too miserable, so I shouted to my boss that we were superior to young people, who work here. Young people nowadays come late for work and leave early. The company's moral has become corrupted. I never, ever, forgive such young ones make fool of us craftmen just because they are keen on computers.
<Y>   "You fought with them, saying that, didn't you?"
<M>   "I'm quiet usually. When I told my subordinate that our company didn't need such a person who try to take paid holiday fully when everybody is working hard, then my boss said, 'Mr. A, don't be so hard. Time has changed.' I felt disgusted. When we tried to take paid holiday in our days, they fired us instantly."
<Y>   "You want to keep rules and discipline, don't you?"
<M>   "We were given an education just after the war... Young people today wouldn't know that we, age 50s, have raised the economy of this country by our desperate efforts.
Presumably, time has changed, but this present time is owing to us who are being made as fool as an old fashioned by those young ones?"

\<Y\>   "Yes, indeed. But those young people, who only seek their own interest, could be the same as people, who sacrificed themselves for their hard work. By the way Mr. A, did you often have a high fever when you were a little?"

\<M\>   "Yes. I had a convulsion due to a fever, and was sent to hospital."

Morning Cuprum \<Support\>   12X x 2 weeks
Night1   Staph   \<Holding anger, an insult\>   200C x 2 days
         Staphysagria also contains a lot of cupper.

2 weeks interval

Night 2 Cuprum \<Constitutional treatment\>   1M x 2 days

Flour-ac
Fl-ac

<Mind>
Materialistic and want to be free all the time. Want to have a lot of lovers (not so much of a sense of guilt). Strong materialistic desires and do anything for obtaining it. Want to steal other people's belongings. They try to get an instant fortune in order to obtain money and a showy life, being immoral and enjoyable. They intend to become an entertainer such as a star or a model. They are extremely cheerful, fear of nothing and are self-satisfaction.
Escaping from responsibilities, committing for matrimonial fraud. Only build up a shallow relationship. Dislike deep and complicated situations. Their ideas change suddenly, and suddenly dislike a person, whom they used to be fond of. They don't treat people as a human and no sympathy to others. No endurance for work is also their character.

<Body>
When fluorine is taken into the body, they become nimble and full of vitality, but after a While, their energy will be depleted, then they become ME, even they are still children.
They hardly go to sleep. Their sleeping hours are short, yet they are still children, and like to eat spicy food. Their body is always warm and sweat a lot. Better from cold-water bathing. Hyperactive. They tend to lack of learning ability. These children are no endurance for both of summer's heat and winter's cold. They have deformities of nails, and pelade.
Diarrhoea by hot food. Keep eating even they are full. They wolf down food and are always hungry. Tongue becomes red and get cracks with tearing pain. Hands and soles are burning hot. Caries, borne problems, tumours grow easily. Swollen gums, weak teeth, chalk like teeth, stripes on teeth. Fluor-ac is effective for the following problems; harmfulness of fluorine (sodium fluoride), bone cancer, ostosarcoma, thyroid problems, enamel on teeth gets disappeared and the teeth get weakened, poikilodentosis, ulitis, kidney disorders, allergy, deformed bones, undeveloped bones.

\<Region\>
Fibrous tissue (vein, skin), Bone, Connective tissue, Mastoid on right side

\<Modality\>

Worse   Hot/Heat (warm room, air, clothes, food, drinks), Night, Alcohol, Sour food, Hunger
Better   Wash in cold water, Open air, Cool, Rapid movement, Nap, Eating

Fluor-ac: Case

12 years old   Boy
Main complaints: M.E. (chronic fatigue syndrome)

He is not able to go to school in ME. He cannot concentrate on and learn at school. Exhausted in crowded places. He's been well known 'Base-ball Boy' till 11 years old before he became like this, he had an abdominal pain suddenly, and started to loose concentration and started to get tired all the time. He is unable to sleep. Shallow sleep keeps him in a bed almost for 10 hours.

<Mother=M> "He wasn't a boy like this... Not even 1 month he was able to go to school in this 1 year. He has no tooth decays or sweet teeth. No fluorine applied on his teeth, I think..."

*If children were abnormally energetic, and sweat a lot with short sleeping hours, that would be a condition, which is incurred shortly after they have taken fluorine and adrenal hormones. However, the energy will be run out in a few years time, then, they will get chronic fatigue syndrome.

1   Fluor-Acid   <Support>   12X x 2 weeks
2   Thuja   <Harmful affect of drugs> 200C x 2 days

He became rebellious to his parents. He started to be able to go to school more often, but still in flattened most of the time. He had slight fevers all the time, while he was taking the remedies.

Morning Selenium   <Support>   12X x 1 bottle (approx. 33 pillules)
Night 1   Fluor-acid   <Constitutional treatment>   200C x 2 days

2 Weeks interval

Night 2   Carcinosin   <Miasm treatment>   1M x 2 days

Iodum
Iod.

<Mind>
Restless. Feel insecure if they keep being quiet. They are urged to move, and get exhausted after the too much moves. They are anxious about their present situation, so they try to be busy for not seeing the situation. No concentration. Always being in conflicts.
Temperamental. Violent. Very forgetful. Driven to over eating. They tell strange jokes often.
They think they are in a fine state. People who were expelled from their country or persecuted in religiously in the past, tend to become Iodum type.

<Body>
Thyroid problems. Over eating, but loose weight. Profuse sweat.
Sweat by little movement. Hyperpnoea. Using up energy. Rough in throat.
Laryngitis. Stuttering and hoarseness. Croupy cough. Gravedo. Rhinitis.
Hardly hear due to blocked ear. Withered breast. Ovarian tumour

<Modality>

Worse   Warm air, Hot air-conditioning, Fasting, Being quiet, Right side
Better Cool open air, Eating

Iodum: Case

25 yeas old   Male (Pakistani)

It is difficult for me to run a relationship with Japanese people. I feel being denied. I feel absent of myself here in Japan as the different culture and the different religion from which I belong to. I think everybody is my enemy. Working harder than anybody else for being accepted. I'm sending 60% of my wages to my family in my country. I suddenly get tempered and have an argument, but my colleagues find me an interesting man. I cannot stop sweating. If somebody stares at me or I stand in front of people, I sweat a lot. My body cannot control temperature well. In Islam, we take a sitting toilet style both for urine and stools. When I do the style for urine, my colleagues tease me, saying "You are always doing Poo.", which I don't like. I don't like Japanese people staring at me. I don't have any friends. I tend to eat too much. I just swallow up without chewing. My body is hot.

<Yui=Y> "Why did you come to Japan?"
<Client=C> "I'm the eldest among 6 brothers, I'm working for my family instead of my father, who hasn't got a job. I came here through a man. I'm working for welding."
<Y>   "Do you enjoy it?"
<C>   "I've never thought if a job is enjoyable or not. If I don't work, my family will be starved to death."
<Y>   "It is hard, isn't it?"
<C>   "I've been like this all the time, so I've never though it is hard."
<Y>   "Do you like Japan?"
<C>   "I haven't been on holiday ever before, just shuttling my apartment and factory, then working for 12 hours a day."
<Y>   "You'd better be honest to your emotions a little bit more. You should take a break sometimes."
<C>   "I don't take a break. When I take a break, I get ill, and it brings back bad memories in the past. I'm fine like this, because I can travel in a dream and I can dream about sea."

<Y>   "Pakistan is at the religious war with India, and has a lot of flood, typhoon and other natural disasters. You didn't have time to look after your spiritual part, did you? All the things you could do there was to live, wasn't it? That's why you are attached to eating. Iodum is the remedy for you. Iodum is also good for immigrants and refugees."

Morning   Nat-m <support>   9X x 1 bottle (approx. 33 pillules) for thyroid and emotional numbness, supporting family.

Night 1   Iodum <support>   12X x 2 weeks
Night 2   Iodum <constitutional treatment> 200C x 2 days

Manganum
Mang.

<Mind>
Strong anxiety and fear. Tearing with smiling. Like to lie down. Tend to go sleep when they have unpleasant and painful things, put things behind, which are supposed to be done. They are always imagining that something bad will be happened. They get better for listening to melancholy music. Dislike happy music. Want to help people, because of being praised by doing so.

<Body>
Tend to lack of oxygen. Tendency of neuralgic problems. Parkinson's disease.
Any part of the body aches by being touched. Fall down forward easily. Pain in knee joints.
Otitis. Tinnitus. Hypoacusis. Thirsty. If they catch cold, pneumonia always follows. Anemia. Pre Menstrual Syndrome (PMS). Menopause. Ostitis. This is an element, which is needed for forming bones

<Modality>

Worse   Cold dump weather, Tomatoes, Feather/dawn kilt, Bend forward
Better   Lying down, Melancholic music

Manganum: Case

12 years old   Girl

She is reluctant to do anything. Pains in her joints. Any hits give her bruises. She is always yawning and being in the clouds. She gets fed up easily when she is given a word by her teacher or parents, then she loses energy, and refuses to go to school. Tends to have diarrhoea by cold foods. She attends girl scout. She loves this activity and never misses it, even it rains. She loves Bach's piano sonata very much.

<Yui=Y> "Does she like tomatoes?"
<Mother=M> "Yes, she does. Even in winter she eats it, but she gets
      diarrhoea soon after
      she eats fresh vegetables."
<Y>   "How about eggs?"
<M>   "Not so much about eggs I think."
<Y>   "If she doesn't eat meat so much, eggs are needed for one in two days at her growing period. 'Free range eggs', which no hormones are fed to chickens, are good for her. Egg contains a lot of manganese, which is being lacked in her."
<M>   "Eggs are in high cholesterol, so I try not to feed her those meat and dairies because it's no good for health. She is taking protein mainly from fish."
<Y>   "Lacking of essential nutrition at growing period disturbs to form strong bones, blood and muscles. Eggs and meats are needed appropriately, although they are not needed to take so much. Some vegetarian parents feed their children vegetables mainly, but I do not recommend the way so much. I think your daughter can grow much bigger. Does she have any hairs on her legs?"
<M>   "Yes, she does. They are thick and bother her, so she shaves them. The hairs are rolled inside and hard to come out."
<Y>   "That is due to lacks of manganese."

Morning Clac-phos 12X x 1 bottle (apporx. 33 pillules)
      <Bone growth, Arthritis>
Night   Manganum 12X x 2 weeks

Palladium
Pall.

<Mind>
Palladium type of people have two side. One is haughty side and the other is weak side, which they easily breakdown to cry. They always want to be shining. Their first aim at a party is to get a centre of attention from others. It could be said 'a syndrome of WANT TO BE PRAISED'. If Palladium type of people are ignored or they think they are ignored, they become hysteric. They used to be in a centre of attention when they were young, so they cannot bear aging, like having wrinkles. They die rushing to cosmetic surgery and aesthetical dental treatment. Mentally they have vanity and become narcissist. They keep behaving very cheerful when they are with other people, but get dead tired after all and weep at home. They tend to be left alone because they think that no one is greater than them.

<Body>
Headache through ear to head and move to other side of the ear.
Right side ovary pain.
Oophorocystosis, Right side disorders (temples, face, eyes, abdomen, ovary, hip)
Skin itchiness. If a part was scratched, another part becomes itchy.

<Region>
Womb, Right ovary, Mind, Right side

<Modality>
Worse Being ignored, Vexation, Humiliation, Standing, Motion
Better Contact, Oppression, Amusement, Rubbing, After sleep, After stools

Palladium: Case

32 years old   Female (Singer)
Main complaints: Ovarian tumour and Thamuria.

I sometimes wet my pants if I don't go to toilet straight away when I feel so. I have suffered from gonorrhoea after I had a sex with a man when I was living in America for studying. Although I am suffering from diarrhoea, there are not so much pains. I have panic attack and am afraid of being alone at night. I wonder, "Why can't people find my value? I sing better, and have better looking than others" while they are getting more famous than I am. I like my job, singing songs, and I love to hear applause after singing. However, I had pain in my tummy, bending doubled, and I collapsed on the stage last time. After the check-up, they found a big ovarian tumour on right side. I'm so afraid of collapsing again. The warts are getting increased on my fingers recently.

Palladium   12X x 2 weeks
Arg-nit   30C x 1 bottle (33 pillules)
           (anytime when she gets panicked)

Platina
Plat.

<Mind>
PLATINA - disappointment or an incident, which they cannot obtain, what they wanted, let them despise other people, their father, theirmother, and their brothers and sisters. And, they tend to leave their family at early age, as if they would rather not be one of suchacontemptible family member. As their pride is high and they make a fool of people, they think people or things are smaller than as they are, although those are actually bigger than them. They have a hatred feeling even towards their loved ones, such as their children and their husband, and they are seized with an impulse to kill them She thinks, "I look like only a house wife, but I really am a chosen existence by God to stand this world as All-Mighty".They are very haughty, and she thinks that people are inferior to her. In fact, Platina type of people become a leader of a group naturally, and are successful. But they look down their subordinates, and their family, handling them roughly. They are narcissists and love themselves the best and admire themselves in a mirror. They are dictators, who want to be shinning all the time. That is why a company director when he/she can't shine and get respect, he/she gets angry and fires employees ruthlessly. Even when a restructuring or achange are needed for an organisation, Platina person is so stubborn and believes him/herself as a great person, then the company will be collapsed eventually.

<Body>
They get vaginitis and they'll be unable to use sanitary pads or tampons. (Tampon is not recommended from a homoeopathic point of view). The vaginal convulsions causes severe dyspareunia that would affect badly to a marital relationship. Tendency of oophrocystosis. Large quantity of tar like black blood at periods. They have PMS (Pre Menstrual Syndrome), are irritable, get depressed, and make a fool of people. They like sex and often change their partner(s), although they have such kind of ovaries and so many vagina problems, because they cannot be satisfied sexually. The other physical problems except for female genital organs, are numbness and pain on scalp, face, coccyx,

and calves. The pain appears slowly and disappears slowly. Tears, stools, and other discharges are cohesive. They feel heaviness while they are resting, and they masturbate a lot. Erections during sleep. They tend to become homosexual. Ailments on right side of the body.

<Modality>
Worse   Deep sorrow, Anger, Insult, Strong emotions, such as sexual excitement, Touch,
Nervous breakdown
Better   Outside, Sunlight, Motion, Stretching body parts, such as extremities

Platina: Case

12 years old   Girl
Main complaints: Temper, Hitting her younger sister

Never obeys, her mother cannot control her. She looks cold-hearted and very haughty.
She wiggles and smirks. She crosses her legs tightly all the time. She touches her clotch.
She had early sexual awakening. Tends to have vaginitis.
Lots of viginal discharges. Defiant attitude towards parents, hitting back, or retorting when she is scolded. Wants to take all her sister's valuables as her belongings. "I don't like this poverty. I'm going to be a company director and will be rich. I want to leave family soon, want to become an adult soon." She does make up, putting gel around her eyes, and gloss on her lips and staring at her in the mirror. When she was 4 years old, her sister was born and mother scolded her severly as a discipline. Her appearance is neater and tidier as a 12 years old girl. Mother also looks smart in shiny white suits with gold frame glasses. Mother has a lot of fillings in her teeth. I asked mother if her uterus system is weak or not. she told me that she had myoma and oohprocystosis and had a surgical operation to take them out. Husband is a factory manager of a watch manufacturer. This girl doesn't have any decayed teeth.

For both mother and girl
Platina 12X x 1 week   Morning and Night

<Yui>   'She has a strong tendency of leaving home at quite early stage. She thinks she is the greatest person, so will start not be able to stand being under parents' control. She will also have sexual tension at early age. She might not be able to concentrate on studying. Platina matches all those problems. If she has a decayed tooth, I recommend to use ceramic or gold as a dental filling even they are relatively expensive. Platina or Palladium would not be good for her.'

Plumbum
Plb.

It could be said that Plumbum 12X massively works for discharging lead from a body, which suffer from plumbism, rather than being used as nutrition absorption.

<Mind>
Oversensitive. Unstable emotions. Depression. Prefer to be alone. Hate people. Desire of killing. Want to stub with using a knife. They think they will be poisoned. Apathetic. Arrogant. Stubborn. Mask (not to show their inside). No concentration. Drops of a memory.

<Body>
Anaemia.
Cramps of legs, muscle twitching with occasional paralysis of muscle and motor nerve.
Parkinson's disease. Chronic nephritis.
Swell of gums. Gums are edged with blue line.
Chronic constipation, and stools are like little balls. Drawing of anus.
Glaucoma.
Old looking and wrinkly skin. Grayish. Evil look as if he/she is criminal.
Chilly extremities.
Pain on the right big toe. Muscle numbness. Loose weight.
Tinnitus and hard of hearing. Corn. Hallux valgus.

<Modality>

Worse   Lying on right side down, Misty, foggy weather, Open air, Excess salivary in high dumpness weather.
Better Bending backward, Bending forward, Oppress strongly, Stretching, Lying

Plumbum: Case

65 years old   Male
Main complaints: Amnesia.

He collapsed due to encephalic thrombosis. After this happened, he has forgotten most of everything of recent events, being paralysis on whole right side, and slur thickly in speaking.
Temperamental. He used to be a chancellor of an university and liked to be surrounded by company, but he got deterioration suddenly, and has started to avoid meeting people as if he is a different person. Before this happened, his family had already problems with him for his forgetfulness. He had not been able to walk so much due to sciatica before he collapsed by thrombosis, but he is getting worse these days.
His hair is so dry and his nails are split. Lead coloured face, having deep wrinkles. He looks empty as senile weak-headed.

Plumbum   12X x 1 week   Morning and Night
Calc-Flour 12X + Silica 12X   x 1 bottle (33 pillules) Noon

Zincum
Zinc

<Mind>
Muddled and slow thinking as if they have fogs in the head. Cannot remember. Weak memory. Not fully developed in brain and nerves. Repeat saying the same thing.
Sleep if they cry. Peevish. Self-pity. They feel as if they commit a crime.

<Body>
Back pain. Pain in bones. Pain in lumbar region. Pain in occiput. Pain in neck. Headache gets worse from wine. Pale face. Aneurysms.
Their legs are restlessness. They feel their legs are heavy.
Itchy skin, especially they feel as if bugs crawling over their skin, especially on a lower half of the body (formication).
Nephrospasis. Dwarfism, problems in growth. Slow in gonad development.
Soreness in extremities, in eyes, and around mouth (Positive-Acraldermatitis).
Dysopia, Dysosmia, Dysgeusia Inappetence, cannot recognise taste or smell.
The stress uses up zinc of internal body, and it leads to have a tendency of becoming Alzheimer.

<Region>
Prostate gland, Retina, Choroid, Semen-Sperm, Diabetes, Muscles, Bornes.

<Modality>

Worse Red wine, Fatigue (exertion of mind and body), After meal, Sweets, 5pm?7pm, Noise, Touch, Suppress eruptions, Suppress discharges
Better Discharges (period starts, diarrhoea, perspiration, etc.), Eating, Scratching, Motion

Zincum: Case

12 years old   Boy
No perseverance. No concentration on studying. It might be too much studying for secondary school entrance exam ahead. He cries with complaining that he has too much to load in his head. No blood circulation to head, having stiff neck all the time and hot. His eye sight is also getting worse.

<Mother=M>   "I want to let him make a success in the exam, but he is getting behind in this situation."
<Yui=Y>   "Any illness, has he had before?"
<M>   "He had a high fever quite often. When he was 9, he got an encephalitis"
<Y>   "How was he at that time?"
<M>   "Weak eyesight and grinding his teeth. He was rolling his head, but all the symptoms were stopped by antibiotic treatment."
<Y>   "Has he got any eczema?"
<M>   "Yes, on his knee. I apply an ointment when he feels itching."
<Y>   "It is wise not to use the ointment. You'd better use Bees wax 'Tu'. It's more natural. So, Mother. You are mentioning that entering to the school is the aim for him. Could you give him some more space after he enters the school?"
<M>   "Of course. But this present is very important".
<Y>   "I understand. Here's a bottle of Zincum for muddled brain, no perseverance nervousness for exam. Please get over these two months with this remedy. Zincum is a No.1 remedy for people, who has to memorise things in repetition. I also prescribe a combination remedy for brains. Ferr-phos of tissue salt, is matched to 'Must be done but can't achieve' very well. Ferr-phos is a support for blood, and it is good for impure blood. When blood is cleaned that makes the head to be clear."
<M>   "Are there any key points for good learning?"

<Y> "Take fresh air in the room. Take a rest and have a sleep when tired. Go to bed early at night, get up early in the morning. It is better to study in the morning, but it might be felt uneasy if he gets up late. Not to eat junk food. Drink coarse tea or water. But Mother, it is important to let him play outside. Too much study at young age tends to give them problems in formation of emotional characteristics with such a twist (Melancholia, Anesthesia).

This is my story; my child's evaluation at school was very good while he's been eating 'Natto'(fermented soy bean). He has perseverance. His younger sister didn't eat it and her level at school was lower middle, but Zincum helped raising her evaluation, and she is now able to sit at a desk longer and calmly than ever before."

HOMOEOPATHY INFORMATION
(as of 22 September 2003)

Homoeopathic Publishing Ltd.
<Headquarters> Homoeopathy Bldg. 1F, 1-14-12 Tomigaya, Shibuya-ku, Tokyo, 151 0063 JAPAN

<Tokyo office> Homoeopathy Japan headquarters bldg., 3-49-13 Nishihara, Shibuya-ku, Tokyo 151 0066, JAPAN

URL http://www.homoeopathy-books.co.jp/
Email info@homoeopathy-books.co.jp

[List of published book]

Mass Immunisation : A point in question
Authour: Trevor Gunn   Translation: Torako Yui
Verification of harmful effects from vaccination. Recommendation to parents who are bringing up their infants.

The Mad Hatter's Tea Party
Authour: Melissa Assilem   Translation: Torako Yui
About remedies, such as tea, caffeine, coffee, sugarcane, and mother's milk. From a viewpoint of women's liberation

Homoeopathy in Japan − a guidebook of homoeopathy 1
Authour: Torako Yui
A definitive comprehensive primer of homoeopathy by Torako Yui Ph.D.Hom.
Complete guide of self-cure. A book for having a good command of basic remedies.

Homoeopathy Guide Book 2 Birth
Authour: Torako Yui and Midwives
A guidebook to support before and after labour

Homoeopathy Guide Book 3 Kids Trauma
Authour: Torako Yui
A manual of remedies for children's diseases and shocks or traumas in a process of children's growth. They are also good for adults to heal their inner child.

Homoeopathy Guide Book 5 Vital Element
Authour: Torako Yui
A guidebook of 12 vital tissue salts remedies and 24 trace elements remedies.

Remedy Note
Authour: John Wallace   Translation: Torako Yui
Materia Medica of 45 remedies, including miasms.
Keynotes of remedies are being expressed by characteristic fonts.

The Spirit of Homeopathic Medicines
Authour: Didier Grandgeorge   Translation: Torako Yui
Introducing approx. 180 remedies. Materia Medica for comprehending the spirits, being showed on remedies.

The Transcript of Lectures 1 Jan Scholten <Elements remedies>
Supervision: Torako Yui
A transcription of Jan Scholten's lecture in Japan. He is a leader of Dutch innovative homoeopathic groups. Epoch making theory, being based on the periodic table.

The Materia Medica of Rajni Satpathy, Indian Homoeopath
Translation supervised by Torako Yui
A simple and clear Materia Medica. An appropriate technical book to people, who are learning homoeopathy.

Systematic Approach In Homoeopathic Theory and Practice
Authour: Mario Boyadzhiev   Translation: Torako Yui
A book, which was systematised unstintingly through his long time experiences.

Antlitz Diagnostik
Authour: Peter Emmrich Translation: Haruki Kumasaka
Translation supervision: Torako Yui
"Face" shows states of our health. We will find which tissue salt is lacked in ourselves by comparing with 11 colour illustrations in the book. An introductory book of vital tissue salts.

Miasms in Labour
Authour: Harry van der Zee   Translation supervised by Torako Yui
To know about labour <the biggest event in a life >, and to overcome it. A book will tell you what is really important to us.

Get Well Soon
Authour: The school of homoeopathy   Translation: Torako Yui
A handbook, very simple and easy to understand. For family's first aid.

The Transcript of Lectures 2 Trevor Gunn <Mass immunisation : A point in Question>
Supervision: Torako Yui
A faithful transcription of Trevor's lectures. Historical two days, when vaccinations' myth was collapsed. Recommendation as a true book to everyone.

Homeopathy A Pictorial Guide
Authour: Judith Scott and Vivienne Rawnsley
Translation: Torako Yui
Easy to look up in cards form. Very useful to keep family member's health.

A Textbook of Dental Homoeopathy
Authour: Dr. Colin Lessell   Translation: Torako Yui

Remedy Note 2
Authour: John Wallace Translation: Torako Yui
61 remedies, including bowel nosodes. For everyone, who wish to make more profound study of homoeopathic remedies.

Schüßler – Salze für Ihr kind
Authour: Thomas Feichtinger / Susana Niedan
Translation Supervision: Torako Yui
Detailed instruction of tissue salts, dealing with children's growth.

A Guide to the Methodologies of Homoeopathy
Authour: Ian Watson   Translation: Torako Yui
Introducing methodologies, which were improved and were developed through the history of homoeopathy. Must be ready by homeopathic college students.

Gesundes Kind – Homoeopathische und naturheilkundliche abwhhrstarkung
Authour: Clementina Rabuffetti Translation supervision: Torako Yui

[Information of Homoeopathy Japan Co.]

Headquarters in Tokyo   Homoeopathy Japan headquarters bldg.,
3-49-13 Nishihara, Shibuya-ku,
Tokyo 151 0066 JAPAN
Tel +81 (0)3 5790 8701
Fax +81 (0)3 5790 8702
URL   http://homoeopathy.co.jp
Email   office@homoeopathy.co.jp

Osaka branch   Homoeopathy Japan Osaka bldg., 3-9-9
Tarumi-cho, Suita city, Osaka 564 0062
JAPAN
Tel +81 (0)6 6368 5352
Fax +81 (0)6 6368 5354

Fukuoka branch   Santen daini bldg. 1F., 3-15-17 Tenjin,
Chuo-ku, Fukuoka city, Fukuoka 810 0001
JAPAN
Tel +81 (0)92 735 7240
Fax +81 (0)92 735 7241

UK branch   Primrose Hill Business Centre, 110
Gloucester Avenue,
Primrose Hill, London NW1 8JA
Tel&Fax +44 (0)20 7209 3734

<Nature of Business>
College The Royal Academy of Homoeopathy Japan (RAH)
Training course (4 years)
    Recognised by the Homeopathic Medical Association (HMA)
    Recognised by the College of Practical Homeopathy (CPH)
    A genuine homoeopathic college for people, who wish to become homoeopaths
Short course for putting 36 basic first remedies into practice(5 times)
    Lectures for people, who wish to have a good command of the 36 remedies.

Homoeopathic consultations (membership basis)
    Lectures about homoeopathy, Practical seminars, Lectures by oversea lecturers
    Homoeopathic network services
    Sales of homoeopathic products (remedy kits, beeswax, etc.)

The Japanese Homoeopathic Centres

In the U.K., many people take homoeopathic consultations for caring their mind and body. In Japan, registered homoeopaths of the JPHMA and the HMA are also opening their consultations in various parts of Japan. In order to live in ourselves as we are, releasing stresses or worries, we wish you to use a homoeopathic centre in your neighbourhood.

The Japanese Homoeopathic Centre

General Supervisor   Torako Yui
URL   http://homoeopathy.co.jp/center_new/
Email   office@homoeopathy.co.jp
NOTE: The consultation is held on membership basis. A person requests a homoeopathic consultation, please join 'Homoeopathy Toranoko-kai'.

Headquarters in Tokyo
Chief: Wataru Katagiri
(Shoko Okamoto, Yoshihiro Nakamura, Asako Hibata, Kuniko Matsumori, Hisae Katayama, Sachiko Koizumi, Etsuko Kamimura, Miki Ishikawa, Kazumori Minami, Mineo Hotta, Chizuru Umaranikar, Yukino Tanaka, Yuka Hamano, Sumiyo Murakami, Yuko Kawase)

Homoeopathy centre headquarters bldg., 2-1-4 Hatsudai, Shibuya-ku, Tokyo 151-0061 JAPAN
Tel +81 (0)3 5352 7750 Fax +81 (0)3 5352 7751

Headquarters in Osaka
Chief: Terue Asano
(Hiromi Hotta, Chieko Takasu, Mari Sou, Makiko Ohno, Noriko Takada, Satoko Yamauchi)

Homoeopathy Japan Osaka bldg., 3-9-9 Tarumi-cho, Suita city, Osaka 564 0062 JAPAN
Tel +81 (0)6 6368 5352   Fax +81 (0)6 6368 5354

Headquarters in Fukuoka
Chief: Seiko Kozonoi
(Setsumi Otani, Katsuki Kishimoto, Ayumi Nakamura, Shoko Takano)

Santen daini bldg. 1F., 3-15-17 Tenjin, Chuo-ku, Fukuoka city, Fukuoka 810 0001 JAPAN
Tel +81 (0)92 735 7240 Fax +81 (0)92 735 7241

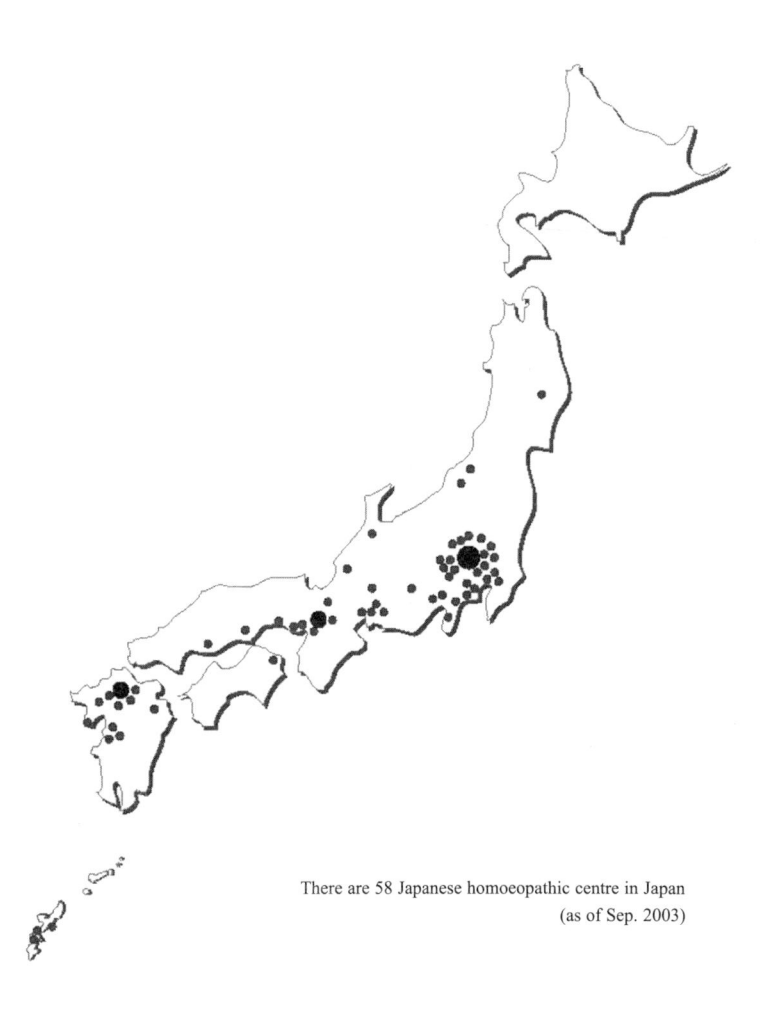

There are 58 Japanese homoeopathic centre in Japan
(as of Sep. 2003)

Iwate Ichinoseki	Mayumi Hongo
Saitama Kawaguchi	Fusako Kawashima
Saitama Higashimatsuyama	Reiko Igarashi
Saitama Fukaya	Machiko Oyama
Saitama Matsubushi	Yasuyuki Yokokawa
Chiba Ichikawa	Hisashi Suzuki
Chiba Funabashi	Yoko Sato
Tokyo Edogawa Minamikoiwa	Keiko Sugimoto, Yumi Suzuki, Yoko Sato
Tokyo Ota Kugahara	Akiko Watanabe
Tokyo Kitashinagawa	Eriko Shimobe
Tokyo Shibuya Harajuku	Yukino Tanaka
Tokyo Sumida Ryogoku	Ayako Tsubota
Tokyo Setagaya Oyamadai	Fumiko Matsushita
Tokyo Setagaya Kyodo	Etsuko Kamimura
Tokyo Chuo Ginza1	Chizuru Umaranikar
Tokyo Chuo Ginza 2	Motoko Watanabe & Yukino Tanaka
Tokyo Nerima Kamishakuji	Noriko Sugahara
Tokyo Hachioji	Nobuko Ueshima

Tokyo Mitaka	Yoshihiro Nakamura
Tokyo Kichijoji	Yoko Minami
Tokyo Musashisakai	Mineo Hotta
Yokohama Tsukuba	Yumi Harada (Inokari)
Yokohama Tsurumi	Chieko Sato
Kawasaki Mizonokuchi	Toshiro Ara
Kanagawa Zushi	Maki Hattori
Kanagawa Chigasaki	Terumi Iwamoto
Kanagawa Hiratsuka	Chihiro Saraya
Kanagawa Tsukimino	Miki Ishikawa
Niigata Agano	Mayumi Inoue
Niigata Nagaoka	Kazumori Minami
Ishikawa Kanazawa	Hiroyasu Mori
Fukui Takefu	Manami Ono
Yamanashi Minami Alps	Kazumasa Fukazawa
Gifu Nagara	Noriko Takada
Shizuoka	Momoko Hara
Nagoya Naka	Kyoko Sakaguchi

Nagoya Mcito	Makiko Ohno
Aichi Toyota	Yasuko Ishigami
Osaka Shin Osaka	Tae Akioka
Osaka Shitenoji	Mari Sou
Osaka Takatsuki	Yuko Teramura
Hyogo Amagasaki	Miyuki Imamura
Hyogo Takasago	Misako Onoe
Okayama Kumayama	Shigemi Matsumoto & Natsumi Matsumoto
Hiroshima Furue	Atsuko Masuda
Fukuoka Yakuin	Yukiko Morishita
Fukuoka Maebara	Setsumi Otani
Fukuoka Kurume	Seiko Kozonoi
Nagasaki Chijiwa	Yumi Miyazaki
Kumamoto Onoue	Msao Shimoda
Kumamoto Hanahata	Taizo Takahashi & Machiko Yamashita
Oita	Shoji Shin
Okinawa Urasoe	Yoko Suzuki

Okinawa Ginowan   Mutsuko Shokita

Okinawa Gushigawa   Nobuko Irei

U.S.A. Pennsylvania   Yumiko Kinoshita